GP ST: Stage 3
Assessment
Handbook

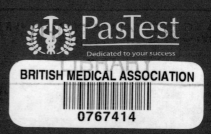

PasTest
Dedicated to your success

GP ST: Stage 3
Assessment
Handbook

Raj Thakkar

BSc (Hons) MBBS MRCGP MRCP (UK)

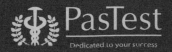

PasTest
Dedicated to your success

© 2008 PASTEST LTD
Egerton Court
Parkgate Estate
Knutsford
Cheshire
WA16 8DX

Telephone: 01565 752000

First Published 2008

ISBN: 1905 635 478

978 1905 635 474

A catalogue record for this book is available from the British Library.

The information contained within this book was obtained by the author from reliable sources. However, while every effort has been made to ensure its accuracy, no responsibility for loss, damage or injury occasioned to any person acting or refraining from action as a result of information contained herein can be accepted by the publishers or author.

PasTest Revision Books and Intensive Courses

PasTest has been established in the field of postgraduate medical education since 1972, providing revision books and intensive study courses for doctors preparing for their professional examinations.

Books and courses are available for the following specialties:
MRCGP, MRCP Parts 1 and 2, MRCPCH Parts 1 and 2, MRCPsych, MRCS, MRCOG Parts 1 and 2, DRCOG, DCH, FRCA, PLAB Parts 1 and 2.

For further details contact:

PasTest, Freepost, Knutsford, Cheshire WA16 7BR

Tel: 01565 752000 Fax: 01565 650264

www.pastest.co.uk enquiries@pastest.co.uk

Text prepared by Carnegie Book Production, Lancaster

Printed and bound in the UK by Page Bros., Norwich, UK

CONTENTS

ABOUT THE AUTHOR

Raj Thakkar, BSc(Hons) MBBS MRCGP MRCP (UK), gained his neuroscience and medical degrees from University College London. During his vocational training in the Oxford deanery, he won the national GP Enterprise Award, registrar division. He currently works as a GP partner in Buckinghamshire, where his special interest is cardiovascular medicine, and as a Hospital Practitioner in Echocardiography. Raj is a freelance writer and GP advisor for several medical magazines.

ACKNOWLEDGEMENTS

The personal perspective sections were contributed by previously successful GP ST applicant, Dr Duncan Rourke, MBBS MA MRCPCh DipOphth. I would like to thank Duncan for his insight and support.

I would also like to thank Hannah Brown, Lily Martin and the team at PasTest for their invaluable advice, encouragement and support in developing this book.

This book is dedicated to my family.

FOREWORD

General Practice is becoming an ever more increasingly popular choice for medical graduates. This is not surprising as Primary Care-led health care becomes a reality with local groups of GPs making Practice Based Commissioning happen. Most general practitioners have control of their working environment, their practice, and relish the opportunity to make their practice a high quality, user-focussed organisation. The new RCGP curriculum and the e-portfolio are leading to a robust and effective professional training to fit young doctors for the many changes in health care over the years to come. The original values and principles that drove the origins of the RCGP have not been lost in the change with patient-centred care and the general practice consultation is as essential to training and day-to-day practice today as they were in the 1960s.

The selection process for General Practice and the GP ST: Stage 3 assessment reflects both those established values together with the needs of 21st century doctors. Throughout 2007 the medical press was full of comments about the failure of the MTAS selection process but there was minimal comment about the effectiveness of the general practice selection system which proved robust. This book builds on that achievement and skilfully guides the reader through the process.

PasTest have an established track record in guiding doctors through their postgraduate exams and in encouraging Raj Thakkar to write for them they have a winning combination. Raj is a practising GP, experienced enough to have a wide field of knowledge but young enough to remember the traumas of taking exams. Raj has used his enjoyment of reading and keeping up-to-date to make the book truly evidence-based but he has also created a very practical book for aspiring applicants to general practice with multiple examples, exercises and scenarios. This is essential reading for any aspiring general practitioner.

Peter Havelock
January 2008

INTRODUCTION

General practice has never been so exciting. The advent of practice-based commissioning (PBC), the new General Medical Services (nGMS) contract and working within a small business make medicine in the community both challenging and rewarding.

Patients present in complex ways and have a number of medical, psychological and social needs. General practitioners (GPs) are charged with the task of teasing out their concerns and managing sometimes quite difficult conditions, as well as looking after their own work–life balance and managing the team with whom they work.

To practise community medicine effectively, a GP requires a number of unique skills, must think in a holistic way and should consult using specialised techniques tailored to the individual patient.

The rewards that general practice has to offer have made the speciality highly competitive. Consequently, a fair and objective entry process has been developed to offer training posts to those most suited to general practice. The General Practice Vocational Training Scheme (GP VTS) application process consists of four stages, some of which are assessments. The competencies tested in the assessments are outlined in the national person specification (NPS).

The NPS outlines the skills and behaviours which examiners are looking for in future GP trainees. Selection methods may vary slightly between deaneries but all will assess candidates against these competencies. It is imperative that each candidate study the specification carefully and consider it while reading this book (see www.gprecruitment.org.uk).

The competencies that are assessed are:

- Empathy and sensitivity: this is the capacity and motivation to take into account others' perspectives and understand their concerns but without over-sensitive involvement. The patient will be treated with understanding using a non-judgemental approach and with appropriate words and actions.

- Coping with pressure: this is the ability to recognise one's own limitations and to seek help where necessary. It requires coping mechanisms to remain under control of difficult situations, maintain the wider focus and respond appropriately when faced with the unexpected.

- Professional integrity: this means having the capacity and motivation to take responsibility and accept challenges, to admit and learn from mistakes and to demonstrate respect and equality of care for all. Patients' needs will be put before one's own when appropriate.

Extract taken from 'GPST: Stage 2 Practice Questions' – Professional Dilemmas.

Candidates are required to be successful in all four stages of the application process to gain a place on a GP training scheme. Stage I considers whether the candidate is eligible to apply for GP training. GMC status and whether the candidate is legally able to work in the UK are checked at this point. Stage 2 is a multiple choice-based assessment taken under examination conditions. Two papers, each of 90 minutes, are designed to test competencies defined under the NPS. Paper 1 tests clinical knowledge whereas paper 2 focuses on professional dilemmas.

Stage 3 is concerned with communication and personal skills, professional integrity and learning. The skills required to pass stage 3 require practice and reflection. Like all things in medicine, there is little room for complacency. Candidates are not expected to have reached the level of a GP registrar, but to demonstrate an appreciation of behaviours and thought processes that a competent GP should possess. These skills are also defined in the NPS (see Table 1). The stage 3 assessment consists of a simulated surgery and may include a combination of an observed group exercise, a prioritisation exercise and a structured interview. These assessments are discussed in separate chapters within this book.

The book guides potential GPs through the stage 3 examination, highlights the behaviours, skills and concepts required to be a successful GP trainee, and offers invaluable practice questions and exercises. Reflective exercises found throughout the book help the reader develop his or her own thought processes and ideas. Time should be spent on these exercises and considered answers should be given to maximise the rewards from the book. The practice questions are similar to those that may appear in the assessments. They should be attempted before reading through the accompanying notes. Chapter 5 summarises a variety of topics that potential GPs should be aware of. These topics may be particularly relevant to the mock consultation and group exercises. Personal experiences of the stage 3 assessment have been kindly contributed by Dr Duncan Rourke and can be found throughout the book.

CHECKLIST FOR STAGE 3 ASSESSMENT

- Check date and time of the assessment
- Check the location
- How will you get there? Have you bought train tickets or do you know where to park?
- Do you need to organise accommodation the night before?
- Have you organised time off work to attend the assessment?
- Have you got a comfortable but smart outfit to wear?
- Remember to bring identification and relevant paperwork as specified by your deanery – this may include:
  - medical degree certificate and current GMC certificate (originals and photocopies)
  - driving licence/passport and/or birth certificate
  - immigration status if required
  - VTR2 forms and/or letters from JCPTGP /RCGP Certification Unit PMETB/Deanery confirming rulings on previous experience (see Appendix A)
  - two structured reference reports from your referees
- Pen
- Watch.

THE INTERVIEW

The majority of deaneries hold a mock consultation, group discussion and prioritisation exercise for the stage 3 assessment. Some, however, may hold an interview. The interview will also be designed to tease out qualities suitable for a career in general practice and virtually any of the skills highlighted in the NPS may be tested.

You should present yourself in a confident manner, maintain good eye contact and avoid fidgeting. As with all interviews, composure, considered responses and honesty are a basic requirement. Clear language should be used. Be prepared to justify any answers that you give to the assessors.

Basic questions are often used to break the ice:
- Tell me about yourself.
- Why would you like to be a GP?
- Where do you see yourself in 5/10 years' time?

Other more directed questions may include:
- Why this scheme?
- Manage a clinical scenario, eg child with asthma, collapse in waiting room.
- Give an example of audit
- Give an example of team involvement that has worked successfully.
- Talk about your own personal development.
- What makes a good GP?
- What qualities do you think a good GP should have?
- What qualities do you have that would make you a good GP?
- How do doctors learn?
- How would you deal with a failing colleague?
- How would you manage a colleague whom you suspect to be depressed?
- How would you deal with a complaint?

- How do you organise your time?
- What do you do to relieve stress?
- How do you break bad news?
- What is patient-centred consulting?
- Why is patient-centred consulting important?

Interview questions may also be based on the topics and practice questions found throughout this book. It is important to practise as may questions as possible, ideally with your peers.

Chapter 1
The Good GP

CHAPTER 1
THE GOOD GP

The GP VTS (General Practice Vocational Training Scheme) assessment aims to identify doctors who have the attributes of a good GP and these are summarised in the national person specification (NPS). The NPS is therefore at the very heart of the entry exams. It is constructive to consider *what* skills and behaviours define a good GP in more detail. Reflecting on *why* a GP should hold these attributes is equally important. Reflection on your own behaviours and changing your practice accordingly is an invaluable aid to learning and personal development (see the NPS).

REFLECTIVE EXERCISE 1

Using the table below, brainstorm what behaviours and skills a GP should have and why.

What skills and behaviours are required?	Why are these important?

As set out in the NPS, a GP is required to have sound breadth and depth of medical knowledge that is up to date. Learning should therefore be a life-long and constant process. GPs should appreciate their limitations, be aware of what they do not know and endeavour to rectify any deficiencies in their knowledge. A lack of awareness of our own deficiencies may lead to clinical mishaps. This concept is described in the Johari window (Luft and Ingham 1955; Luft, 1961, 1969).

Doctors should be aware that learning is not always a passive exercise. Although reading journals and guidelines is important, learning needs may become apparent in a number of different ways.

CHAPTER 1

REFLECTIVE EXERCISE 2

Consider how learning needs may arise by filling in the table below.

What skills and behaviours are required?	Why are these important? (reader to brainstorm)

CHAPTER 1

Learning needs may arise from a number of different sources:
- Known deficiencies
- New guidelines/medical breakthrough
- Course, journal
- General discussion
- A question arising during surgery or a clinical situation you're not sure how to manage (patient's unmet needs and doctor's educational needs – PUNs and DENs – coined by Dr Richard Eve in Somerset (Eve R, 2003))
- Clinical errors
- Audit
- Patients' complaints.

How GPs learn is equally important:
- Personal reading: journals, textbooks
- Internet resources, learning websites
- Courses
- Lectures
- Reflection on your own practice
- Significant event analysis.

It is important to know where to find reliable medical information, to be able to appraise it and to consider what and how to apply new knowledge to your own patients.

The consultation is at the heart of general practice, and it takes years to refine the art of consulting. GPs tend to have a short period of time to consult with each patient. During those 10 minutes, they have to elicit a directed history, examine appropriately and formulate a management plan that is acceptable to the patient. A patient's concerns have to be addressed so that the patient leaves satisfied that the doctor is acting in his or her best interests. The consultation must be conducted with empathy and sensitivity, using appropriate language that the patient understands. When managing patients, a number of issues may need to be considered: legal, ethical, safety, society, cost, etc. Doctors should be aware of wider issues in order

CHAPTER 1

to bring the situation to an appropriate conclusion. These skills are required under the NPS.

A GP may see many patients during an average working day. It is imperative that each patient be given high-quality health care. Some patient encounters may be stressful, intense and frustrating whereas others will be satisfying and fulfilling. Many of these consultations will generate paper work. In addition, dozens of letters and test results will need to be reviewed on a daily basis and home visits will need to be dealt with. It is important for all doctors to be organised, to prioritise their work and to deal with tasks efficiently.

Housekeeping is a concept described in Neighbour's model of consultation (Neighbour 2004). Doctors must learn to look after themselves, manage stress, recognise when they need help and know where to find it. Support may be found from colleagues, your own GP, the local medical committee (LMC) and agencies such as the British Medical Association (BMA). Other members of the health-care team may be stressed for a number of reasons; we should be aware of this, consider why they may be feeling that way and offer appropriate support.

Although GPs spend much of their day working independently, the success of a practice depends very much on teamwork. GPs should consider the views of all members of the multidisciplinary team and be able to negotiate effectively.

Probity encompasses a number of issues surrounding professional integrity. Honesty when at work, performing research, the receipt of gifts, relationships with patients and issues surrounding practice finances are all examples. The GMC have clear guidelines on these and many other issues.

Being a good doctor includes, but goes far beyond, being clinically sound. Honesty, never cutting corners, knowing your limits, behaving appropriately, looking after yourself and others, and being able to justify your actions are principles that all doctors may want to consider. The stage 3 assessment may consider all of these issues and more.

Chapter 2
Mock Consultation

CHAPTER 2
MOCK CONSULTATION

The simulated consultation is usually conducted with an actor and observed by examiners. It tests virtually all the criteria set out in the national person specification (NPS), particularly clinical knowledge and expertise, empathy and sensitivity, communication skills, and conceptual thinking and problem-solving. Before the exercise, you will be given written instructions outlining the scenario. The actor will also have instructions to bring out particular issues during the consultation.

You will be faced with one of many types of scenario. The exercise can be nerve-racking but, as with all exams, preparation and practice will get you through. Role-playing with colleagues and trying these techniques on real patients will make stage 3 a joy. When role-playing, it is helpful for colleagues to critique your effort, giving constructive feedback.

SIMULATED SURGERY MARKING SCHEME

The mock consultation is marked using set criteria in order to standardise the assessment. Both the observer and the actor are asked to give their feedback and their scores are combined to provide an overall rating for the simulation.

The criteria are divided into three categories, communication skills, empathy and sensitivity, and problem solving.

Communication skills: high marks will be awarded if the patient (actor) feels you communicate in an effective way overall and if problems are explained using clear and appropriate language. Analogies, diagrams and leaflets are examples of adjuncts that may be used to augment effective communication. Adjusting your language to a level the patient understands is important. You should ensure both you and the patient have clarity about what the problems are and what the management is. Asking open rather than closed questions score highly. Patients should feel enabled to tell you what their concerns are. Looking interested and concerned, with good eye contact, suggests to the examiners you are genuine in your care for the patient in front of you.

Empathy and sensitivity: The patient will give you high marks if they feel you understand their feelings, situation and concerns. They should feel confident that their concerns are being addressed. Assessors will be looking to see if you're interested in your patient. You may be genuinely interested, but if the patient doesn't feel it and the assessor doesn't see it, you will not score highly. A judgemental approach, making false assumptions and behaving in a dictatorial way will be frowned upon. You should be seen to create a positive atmosphere which is relaxed and you should earn your patient's trust.

Problem solving: You should demonstrate you are able to identify the patient's concerns and take an appropriate history for each one. Each problem may require appropriate investigations, treatment and follow-up that is suitable to the patient. The assessors will be impressed if you manage to identify the salient problems, think widely and are open minded. Aim to prioritise the patient's problems and deal with each one in turn. The consultation should be structured and time managed appropriately.

CONSULTATION MODELS

There are a number of published consultation models that GPs use when managing patients. An appreciation of these consulting styles is required for stage 3 rather than an in-depth knowledge. GPs consult in a patient-centred way, that is, involving the patient in their illness, encouraging them to express their concerns and involving them in the management, rather than the more traditional doctor-centred style of clerking. Two of the models are summarised below. The choice of the model used is dependent on the doctor's style and preference as well as on patients and what their problems are. There are common themes among many of the consultation models.

THE NEW CONSULTATION
(PENDLETON ET AL. 2003)

Task 1

To understand the reasons for the patient's attendance. Consider the patient's problems including cause and effect, and what their ideas are about its causes and management. What concerns do they have? What are their expectations?

Task 2

Achieve a shared understanding, by taking the patient's perspective into account. What is their understanding of the problem and its management?

Task 3

To enable the patient to choose an appropriate action for each of their problems. Discuss and choose management options with patient.

Task 4

To empower the patient to manage the problem. Ensure that the patient has the ability to manage the illness. Agree the roles of the patient and doctor. Agree on appropriate follow-up.

Task 5

To consider other problems. Are there ongoing issues that need addressing? Are there risk factors that need addressing?

Task 6

To make appropriate use of time during the consultation and in the longer term.

Task 7

To establish or maintain the doctor–patient relationship that helps to achieve the other tasks.

CHAPTER 2

THE INNER CONSULTATION

(NEIGHBOUR 2004)

- Connect: establish a trusting doctor–patient relationship.
- Summarise: active listening, ensure that the patient understands the doctor and the doctor understands the patient.
- Handover: formulation of management plan and give patient responsibility to execute treatment.
- Safety-net: criteria given to patient when to seek medical advice.
- Housekeeping: looking after yourself.

REFLECTIVE EXERCISE 1

It is important to reflect on why you think a consultation should be tested in the exam.

The simulated consultation is designed to show off your consultation skills rather than to scrutinise your clinical acumen. Nevertheless, glaring clinical mistakes should be avoided and the examiners will expect a safe standard of medical practice. All doctors will come across situations that test their clinical abilities. It is far safer to explain that you need to check something out, discuss the situation with a colleague or refer for further advice than to muddle through dangerously.

The interaction between the doctor and patient is pivotal to a successful outcome. GPs consult in a very different style to hospital practitioners. There are a number of reasons for this. Consultations in the community tend to be time limited – GPs spend approximately 10 minutes on each consultation. Running behind in a busy surgery may be stressful for GPs and frustrating for patients. Patients may offer hidden agendas in the community with far more subtle cues than in hospital medicine.

During a consultation, the GP may have to take a history, examine the appropriate system(s), and diagnose and formulate a management plan for each of the patient's presenting features. In many cases the consultation is a follow-up or the GP knows the patient very well, in which case a full history is not always required. Nevertheless, the time must be used efficiently in order to reach the desired outcome. There is little time to use the traditional 'hospital style' of clerking. GP registrars tend to be allocated 30 minutes per consultation when they first begin their training. It is considered important to develop the right consultation skills first before trying to fit the whole process into 10 minutes.

It may be possible to get by in general practice by simply dealing with the medical problem at hand, ie asking relevant, but perhaps closed, questions, telling the patient the likely diagnosis, explaining what investigations are required and giving a treatment plan. This doctor-centred style of consulting is, however, often very unsatisfying for the patient.

CHAPTER 2

REFLECTIVE EXERCISE 2

Can you think of any reasons why patients may find doctor-centred consultations unsatisfactory?

The assessment is meant to be as life-like as possible. In everyday practice, the manner in which you greet the patient and develop any rapport may make or break the consultation. A welcome gesture or handshake will put the patient at ease. You should introduce yourself so that the patient knows who you are and your designation. Clearly, your approach must be tailored to the individual patient. A light-hearted welcome may not be appropriate for a patient who enters your consulting room in tears. An intrusive desk between the patient and the doctor can be a barrier to a sensitive consultation. The patient's chair should be to the side of your desk.

A number of open questions should be used in your initial statement. By using open questions and giving the patient an opportunity to speak, much of the history can be elicited. Patients should not feel rushed but enabled to explain their concerns. Their illness should be considered in a social context and patients should be enabled to express their own ideas about their diagnosis, its causes and treatment options. You should establish the effect of the illness on the patient's life and any concerns that they have.

Consider the following consultation:

Doctor: So you have had stomach pains since this morning?

Patient: Yes.

Doctor: Where does it hurt?

Patient: Down here. [Pointing to right iliac fossa.]

Doctor: Is it sharp or dull?

Patient: Sharp.

Doctor: Does it hurt when you pass urine?

Patient: No.

Doctor: Are you constipated?

Patient: No.

You can see that the dialogue is monotonous and does not give the patient much opportunity to express him- or herself. Compare it with the patient-centred consultation below:

Doctor: So you have had stomach pains since this morning. Tell me more about that?

Patient: It woke me up. It's really sharp [pointing to right iliac fossa], especially when I move. I couldn't even eat breakfast. The pain is just getting worse. My partner thought it might be a urine infection but it doesn't hurt when I pass urine. Is it my appendix?

Doctor: You may well be right! I just want to check out a couple of points if that's ok. Can you tell me when your last period was?

Patient: I don't have periods; I had a coil a few months ago.

The second consultation is more like a flowing conversation, engaging the patient and eliciting much of the history with an opening statement. As the consultation progresses, closed questions may well need to be asked.

Patients see their GP for a number of reasons. Take the example of a sore throat. It may be that the patient simply wants treatment for an upper respiratory tract infection and nothing more. Other reasons for consulting should nevertheless be explored. The patient may be hoping that the doctor will link the sore throat to smoking habits and then offer help on quit strategies rather than a lecture on the dangers of smoking from 'a doctor who isn't interested'.

If a good rapport is struck and the patient feels at ease, he or she may feel enabled to offer a cue for the doctor to pick up on. For example, he or she may ask if having a sore throat is a sign of being run down. If a doctor is *actively* listening to the patient, they could explore this comment, checking out whether the patient is anxious, stressed or even depressed. Patients may be more subtle in the cues that they offer and look sad or be reluctant to leave the consulting room, hoping

CHAPTER 2

that the doctor may suggest 'You look sad. Is everything ok?' or 'You seem worried. Is there anything on your mind?'. Delving deeper, the patient may have other concerns about the sore throat. The patient may be worried that, if it is a bacterial tonsillitis, her spouse, who is on chemotherapy, may be at risk of infection. Her uncle may have been recently diagnosed with throat cancer and the patient may be worried that she has throat cancer too. It is important to be aware that patients may have concerns related to their symptoms that you may not think about.

Checking whether a patient has any questions or concerns will make the patient feel valued, listened to and, above all, their anxieties will be addressed. If the doctor is not actively listening, ignores or misses a cue, a serious medical condition may be missed and the patient can feel frustrated and dissatisfied. Cues are often difficult to pick up on and eliciting hidden agendas features in higher-level exams. It is important, however, to be aware that cues exist and to appreciate that patients do not always offer their worries on a plate.

Once patients' concerns have been addressed, they may want to know how long the illness will last, if it is dangerous, contagious, etc. Patients often want to know what to expect from their illness and doctors should not assume patients' knowledge. We may offer them medication and usher them out of the door, knowing full well that they will get better, but patients do not know that. They will leave the consulting room frustrated with more questions than answers. How will they know when to come back if they do not know what the course of the illness is likely to be? Managing patients' expectations empowers them to help themselves. It is not always possible or appropriate to admit patients about whom we are unsure. Giving them a series of guidelines to help them manage their own illness and when to seek further medical advice is good practice. This is known as safety netting. In this way, patients feel empowered and leave the consulting room satisfied.

Nowadays patients are far more aware of their own health than they used to be. It is not unusual to be presented with the latest

NICE (National Institute for Health and Clinical Excellence) guidelines, newspaper cuttings or reams of information from the internet. This is part of the reason why patients should be involved in the management of their condition. Shared management makes patients feel involved and listened to by their doctors. Take, for example, antibiotics and sore throats. Some doctors may assume that a patient wants antibiotics. Of course, it may be true that the patient has tonsillitis, is feverish, feels unwell and desperately wants penicillin. On the other hand, the patient may not want antibiotics, but reassurance that it is not cancer or that it is likely to get better with analgesics. Sharing management with patients is therefore an important part of patient-centred consulting. A simple way to share management is to give patients all the possible treatment options, discussing the pros and cons of each one, so that they can make an informed decision.

During the consultation, it is important to check that you have understood what patients have said by summarising what they have said back to them:

> 'So just to recap, you've been having abdominal pain for
> two days, it is in the upper right part of your "stomach", is
> sharp and it comes and goes. Have I got that right?'

Conversely, it is important to check that patients have understood what you have said by asking them or by summarising and reiterating your point. Recapping the management plan is also one of many ways to round off the consultation.

To keep the patient fully involved in the consultation, many doctors sign-post, which is explaining to the patient the direction of the consultation:

> 'If it's ok with you, I'll ask you a few more questions and
> then examine you. I will need to examine your hips if
> that's ok. Sometimes a painful knee is related to problems
> in the hip itself. We can then decide how best I can treat
> you. So tell me more about your knee symptoms ... .'

CHAPTER 2

Patient-centred consulting makes the patient feel at ease, listened to, valued, involved and satisfied that the doctor has taken an interest. Of course, a good consultation does not replace, but complements, the practice of safe medicine. A GP must consider the illness in a social context, ie how it affects the patient's and the patient's family's life. Empathy is crucial.

GP registrars are tested on patient-centred consultation models at MRCGP level. At stage 3, you are not expected to be able to consult fluently using this style of consulting, but to show an appreciation of the concepts and follow the basic principles of patient-centred consulting.

CHAPTER 2

SUMMARY

Reasons why patients may present to their GP:
* Physical complaint
* Hidden agenda
* Mental illness
* Social problems
* Worried well
* Follow-up for chronic illness
* Follow-up from a previous consultation
* For personal gain
* To complain
* To enquire about others
* To express concern about others.

Ways in which patients may present:
* Explicit: 'I feel depressed'
* Hidden agendas: doctor may need to search for the underlying agenda – 'Do stressed people get sore throats?'
* Cues: patients may offer the doctor a cue – 'You look worried, you seem low'
* Somatisation
* Angry
* Sad
* Inappropriate.

Style of consulting:
* Make the patient feel at ease and welcome appropriately; introduce yourself.
* Don't sit across the table from the patient if possible.
* Consider what patients think is going on, their concerns (worried if they have cancer) and any expectations about how the condition may be investigated, treated and the clinical course for each condition.

CHAPTER 2

- What does the patient know already about the issue being discussed?
- Actively listen. Are there cues for hidden agendas?
- Check that you have understood what the patient has tried to say, perhaps by summarising back to him or her.
- Involve patients in their own health; share clinically appropriate management options.
- Safety net.
- Follow up appropriately.
- Regularly check if the patient has understood what you have said. Your language should be tailored to the individual. Can you offer leaflets or websites for the patient to refer to, eg www.patient.co.uk?

CONSULTATION MNEMONIC

WISSSH:

W Welcome patient, make him or her feel at ease

ICE What are the patient's ideas, concerns and expectations?

S Summarise, check that you have understood patient and that the patient has understood you

S Share management, give patient the options and agree a management together

S Safety net

H Health promotion, discuss patient's lifestyle.

' For the role-played consultation, I was observed discussing an equivocal stomach ulcer biopsy report with a "patient". Before the consultation I was given time to read the histology report and some brief notes about the patient. The consultation was not strictly time limited and I was advised that I should finish when I thought it appropriate. I took my time reading the information to ensure I had the facts in my head, and pointedly arranged the chairs in what I considered a non-confrontational pattern.

Before the day, I had done some reading online about "the medical consultation" and the various models that break down the interview into component parts. I would strongly recommend doing this as it gave me some sense of control over the process, and a confidence that I was probably ticking the observer's boxes as the consultation progressed. Developing a rapport is obviously of paramount importance, and that should probably start with a friendly introduction, handshake and eye contact with the "patient". No doubt we are judged on how this part of the consultation goes, and I think it's worth giving prior thought to the precise words you might use by way of greeting, lest you find yourself gabbling something overly paternalistic, casual or cringe worthy.

Things that I felt went well during my consultation include the following: being seen to let the patient talk, establishing the patient's agenda early on, exploring wider issues such as family, getting a feel for how the patient was dealing with things emotionally with questions like "How do YOU feel about that?", registering my sympathy when appropriate, acknowledging the patient's difficulties, and ending with a clear, mutually agreed plan about what would happen next for the "patient". I would add that it probably does not hurt to sign-post these elements of the consultation to the observer .... '

Dr Duncan Rourke

Stage 2 GP VTS

PRACTICE SCENARIOS

It is worth practising these scenarios with one colleague playing the patient and others critiquing. In the assessment, you will be given time to make notes. As such, space has been provided below each scenario to brainstorm your ideas. Notes have then been included with each scenario. You may well think of other points in addition to these. The notes accompanying each scenario are by no means complete but may stimulate further discussion. More practice questions may be found in Chapter 6.

SCENARIO 1: PATIENT WITH CHEST PAIN

Martin, a 64-year-old man who smokes, attends your clinic having experienced exertional chest pains over the past few weeks. He seems worried. You are asked to see the patient and make an appropriate management plan. Assume, for the purposes of this exercise, that there are no abnormal findings on clinical examination. He is currently pain free.

CHAPTER 2

NOTES

- It is important to keep in mind the possible differential diagnoses when talking to the patient, eg CHD, thromboembolic disease, neoplastic disease, dyspepsia, musculoskeletal.
- You could ask the patient closed questions:

  Where is the pain? Is it sharp or dull? What makes it worse?
- It is more patient-centred to say:

  'Tell me about it … tell me about your pains … tell me more … go on … ?'

  and let the patient speak. As with many presenting complaints, much of the history can be gleaned using open-ended questions.
- While the doctor may be concerned about ischaemic heart disease or lung cancer, the patient may have an entirely different concern, COPD, for example, after seeing his best friend die from it. Exploring the patient's ideas and what he thinks is going on is important.
- The patient may be anxious so it is vital to explain what you think may be going on in appropriate language and to check that the patient understands. Only then can the patient agree or disagree to go for further tests. Martin's anxiety may be so high that he does not seem to be taking in what you are saying. Options in this case may be to acknowledge his anxiety and explore the reasons why Martin is so agitated. If clinically safe, you may offer to see him at the end of clinic once he has had the chance to settle down. Does he have a history of anxiety? Is this cardiac neurosis?
- He may be in denial and not want further intervention. Reasons for this include genuine disinterest in intervention and consulting to please his wife, depression, poor health expectations for himself or total fear of serious pathology.
- Checking out the patient's knowledge and informing the patient of what ischaemic heart disease is, what the causes are, what investigations and treatments may be available are imperative to get the patient on board with further management.
- Asking what Martin's views are on smoking rather than lecturing him on its dangers may prove fruitful. He may already want to quit but does not know how. See 'cycle of change' in relation to addiction (p58).

SCENARIO 2: THE ANGRY RELATIVE

Jason is a patient of yours who you have been treating for
depression. He hasn't improved on the antidepressant that
you prescribed recently. He has been performing badly
at work and is at risk of being sacked. Jason's wife, Claire
attends your clinic and is angry that his antidepressants
haven't worked. You are to manage Claire's anger
appropriately.

NOTES

- It is not unusual for relatives to attend with their loved ones. This may be for a number of reasons. Frustration, as in this case, is a common scenario. Another is where the patient is unlikely to remember all the details of the consultation, perhaps someone with dementia.

- Claire's anger should not be ignored. Consent should be sought from Jason before any further conversation takes place between you and his wife. Without consent, the specifics of his case must remain confidential. Of course, there are many general points about depression that can be discussed. It may be worth finding out what she knows/what he has told her so far.

- Acknowledgement of her anger is a good way to diffuse the situation. Demonstration of empathy, suggesting that it must be difficult and frustrating for her, may prove fruitful and pacify her.

- Perhaps explore her ideas about what depression is, what she thinks Jason is experiencing, what treatments are available and what course the illness takes. She may not realise that antidepressants take at least 2 weeks before they start to work. Be careful not to be patronising.

- She is angry and may have specific concerns that need to be addressed. Perhaps she suspects that Jason is unhappy in their marriage, or maybe even having an affair and she wants information. If her concerns are not dealt with, she may continue to feel frustrated. She may fear that he will deteriorate and not be able to work or he may be violent; Claire may be concerned that he will harm himself or their child.

- She may have other treatment options in mind. It is worth asking them both about this and discussing the pros and cons of each modality.

CHAPTER 2

SCENARIO 3: THE POORLY ADHERENT PATIENT

Angus is a 46-year-old businessman with diabetes and hypertension. He has come to see you in a routine diabetic clinic. You notice on his electronic records that he has not been collecting his repeat prescriptions. His HbA1c (glycated haemoglobin) has been creeping up over the last 18 months and is now too high at 10.1%.

You are to approach the subject of poor adherence with Angus and consider ways to help with his medication.

NOTES

- It is important to gain good rapport with the patient and gain his trust.

- Consider asking open questions first, such as 'How's your diabetes? … How do you think your diabetes is going? … '

- This approach may provide you with valuable information about his knowledge base, motivation and understanding. If he does not know much about diabetes, it is important to explain more about the condition. Given that you have asked him an open-ended question, he may admit to not taking his medication.

- He may not have been taking his drugs for a number of reasons – denial, depression, side effects, fear of side effects, he may want to defeat diabetes through lifestyle or other means, he may not understand the significance of omitting to take his pills. Exploring his concerns and addressing these issues are vital.

- If he does not offer you inroads into questioning about his adherence, perhaps discussing the HbA1c result is a good start. Again, you ought to ask him if he understands the significance of the test. Then offer explanations as to why it may have increased, poor adherence being a cause.

- What other drugs has he not been taking?

- Formulate and agree a management plan that he is happy with. It is important that he understands the risks of poor adherence. Perhaps make a management 'contract'.

- Appropriate follow-up, perhaps with a repeat blood test and blood pressure, should be arranged.

- Health promotion issues should be discussed: weight; is he a smoker?

SCENARIO 4: BREAKING BAD NEWS

Nicola is a 47-year-old teacher who was referred to the surgical team with a 2-month history of bleeding per rectum. Both her sister and her father have had surgery for bowel cancer. Unfortunately her father died recently. Nicola had a colonoscopy 2 weeks ago and has come to get the results of a lesion that was biopsied. Your consultant has been called away urgently and you have been asked to break the news that she has bowel cancer. She has come to clinic with her partner, Robert.

CHAPTER 2

NOTES

- Doctors often feel uncomfortable when they have to give bad news. Greeting the patient in an excessively happy demeanour is inappropriate.
- It is best not to assume knowledge or that the patient is going to take the news badly. Some patients are philosophical whereas others are devastated by such news.
- Checking out what happened at the last consultation and to confirm why the patient has attended is a good start and will allow you to assess the patient's background knowledge. It will also confirm that you have the right patient. She may at this point ask 'Have I got cancer, doctor?'
- It is worth trying to establish how much detail the patient wants to receive. Do not assume that patients want to be wrapped in cotton wool or to be told the blunt facts. Perhaps ask the patient what their fears are.
- The build-up to breaking bad news should not be overdone; the patient may become agitated.
- The bad news should be delivered with empathy, in simple English but without being patronising.
- Give the patient time; a short silence is appropriate.
- Check her understanding.
- Offer her and her partner a chance to ask questions; perhaps they will want some time alone. It is likely that they will want to know what happens next.
- There may be questions that you cannot answer. Be honest if you do not know.
- The couple may be angry that the consultant was not present, it does no harm to apologise.

SCENARIO 5: THE SAD PATIENT

Amy is a 19-year-old student whom you have known for many years. She presents to clinic with frontal headaches for a few days. You notice that she looks unhappy and stressed. You are to take a history and explore any underlying causes. Assume for the purposes of the assessment that her neurological exam and blood tests are normal.

NOTES

- General practice allows the GP to get to know their patients and changes in physical or mental functioning may be apparent.
- She presents with an obvious cue, looking sad.
- It may be appropriate to take the cue early, suggest that she does not look happy and wait for a reply. You may want to link this to her headache, suggesting that one of the most common causes is stress and ask if everything is ok.
- You should not omit to rule out important organic causes of headaches.
- She should be assessed for depression, eating disorders, risk of self-harm, drugs and alcohol, and psychosis if appropriate.
- A social history is important here. What are her home circumstances? Are there relationship or financial issues? Perhaps she is being bullied at work or is fearful of starting university.
- Is she worried about a brain tumour?

SCENARIO 6: A COLLEAGUE'S MISTAKE

Rebecca, aged 25 years, attends your clinic for a routine pill check. You look through her notes and see that her last smear, which was 6 months ago, was inadequate and another smear was recommended. The result was overlooked by her usual doctor and Rebecca was unaware that the smear had to be retaken. The pill check is normal and you now need to explain the oversight to the patient.

NOTES

- This situation is a very real possibility. Human errors unfortunately happen.
- The patient may have had her repeat smear elsewhere, perhaps privately. She may have also had it at the clinic but, for some reason, there is no documentation. Asking Rebecca when and where her last smear was taken is a reasonable question.
- Honesty is the best option. She should be told about the oversight. Give her time to gather her thoughts, and explore her concerns.
- An apology should be made and an appointment for a smear offered.
- She may become angry. Acknowledge this; understanding her anger demonstrates empathy. Is there anything else that she would like you to do? Offering to look into why it happened and holding a meeting may be enough (critical event analysis, see p85).

OTHER POINTS TO CONSIDER

- Explaining what happened to the doctor who missed the result.
- What happens if the repeat smear is abnormal?
- After holding the critical event meeting, are there any systems that can be put into place to ensure that this does not happen again? Have there been any other oversights, eg blood tests? What about other smears? Has that doctor been making other mistakes? Does that doctor need support?
- The patient may make an official complaint.

CHAPTER 2

Chapter 3
Group Exercise

GROUP EXERCISE

We spend much of our time in general practice working independently. Many of the non-clinical decisions that we make, however, are made as a team. Our views, wants and actions can have a huge impact on our colleagues and patients. The team task assesses how the candidate interacts with his or her peers. A number of skills from the national person specification (NPS) are tested, in particular, empathy and sensitivity, communication skills, organisation and planning, managing others and team involvement, and professional integrity.

Groups of three to four candidates are observed for 10–20 minutes while they discuss the issue presented to them. Each member of the group has 20 minutes to read through an individualised brief before the discussion. It is important to use the preparation time wisely and brainstorm key issues that are relevant to the topic. Participants are sometimes asked to play different members of the multidisciplinary team and this will be mentioned in the brief. There will usually be one observer per candidate, assessing a number of different skills and attributes.

A variety of different tasks may be asked of the group. A decision may need to be reached about a particular issue or a generalised discussion may be required. To debate issues with strong and logical arguments, an appreciation of concepts and topics is required. As such, subjects including audit, significant event analysis, management of change, practice-based commissioning (PBC) and out-of-hours (OOH) provision are covered later in the book. Candidates may be expected to consider wider issues pertaining to a given scenario such as legal aspects, ethical viewpoints, communication, safety, training, time, resources and effects on the local community, staff, patients and public.

REFLECTIVE EXERCISE

Can you think of some examples where team decisions are required?

There are an infinite number of subjects that may require discussion and various members of the multidisciplinary team may be invited. Topics of discussion may or may not be directly related to patient care. Many GP practices will have weekly meetings where many decisions are made. Examples include:

- Rotas
- Annual leave
- Implementing new guidelines
- Dealing with finances
- The Christmas party
- Purchasing new equipment
- Developing a chronic disease clinic
- Handling a receptionist who is rude to the patients
- Adverse clinical events
- Introduction of a practice website
- An online booking system for the practice
- Redecoration
- A new telephone system
- Should you teach medical students at the practice?

One of the participants will need to start the discussion off, which may be nerve-racking when being watched, but reflects leadership and confidence. Each candidate, however, should be enabled to summarise his or her brief and initial views before the debate gets into full swing. A leader may naturally evolve as the discussion progresses. Leadership skills are assessed by the examiners, including giving others an opportunity to speak and considering their views, politely keeping the group focused on the subject rather than going off on a tangent and keeping the discussion moving forward finally to reach a conclusion. All parties should ideally be in agreement with the decision-making process and the final outcome. Try to reach an agreement in the allotted time.

Some of the marks are allocated to the content of the discussion. Candidates will be expected to think widely, and to acknowledge that there are a number of factors that need to be taken into consideration when debating the issue at hand and that people can be affected in different ways.

CHAPTER 3

Clear comments that are backed up by robust arguments will score highly. It is important to offer your views but also to listen actively, and give others a chance to respond and share their own views with the group. Marks will therefore be awarded for active participation in the discussion but also for allowing and encouraging others to contribute. If another candidate's point is poorly understood, it is far better to ask for clarification than to make a false interpretation. By the same token, summarising your own points, if complex, may impress the examiners.

The examiners will be keen to observe negotiation skills, the ability to appreciate another person's point of view, the willingness to compromise and a calm temperament. Behaving in a dictatorial, narrow-minded or confrontational way will be frowned upon, as it would in everyday life.

Some members of the discussion group may be quiet and they may lose points for this. On the other hand, monopolising the conversation, not inviting quiet members of the group to speak and arrogance are likely to upset the examiners. People may be quiet for many reasons including a lack of confidence, frustration, anger and distraction (eg they feel unwell).

Non-verbal cues are also considered by the examiner. All participants should look attentive and interested rather than apathetic or aggressive.

'For the team task I joined three other applicants and four observers in a room. We were asked to consider four imaginary junior doctor colleagues who each had a particular problem relating to their medical work. We were told to come up with a plan for how we might resolve their problems and were explicitly asked to rank the four problems in order of seriousness. The four imaginary junior doctors were: a colleague who was depressed and had recently made potentially life-threatening drug prescription errors that were fortunately noticed by nursing staff, the colleague who was thought to have an abusive relationship out of work and for whom work standards were slipping, a hard-working colleague who continued to self-prescribe steroids for asthma in spite of previous warnings, and an arrogant colleague who created division and problems among fellow staff. As a team we all went to great lengths to be simultaneously good at listening and contributing. We all nodded encouragingly at appropriate moments and gave each other the opportunity to take the stage and have our say. I think the smart game player will also bring some personality to the table to make themselves stand out if the opportunity presents itself. In other words, do not be afraid to be yourself. I think we did well as a team in that we established a "duty of care" to our patients' safety as the driving principle in deciding how we rank our troubled imaginary colleagues. With this principle in mind (and reiterated just in case the observers had not heard us all say it four times) we worked fairly swiftly towards an agreed plan of action … . '

Dr Duncan Rourke

Stage 2 GP VTS

PRACTICE SCENARIOS

It is worth practising these scenarios with one colleague playing the patient and others critiquing. In the assessment, you will be given time to make notes. As such, space has been provided below each scenario to brainstorm your ideas. Notes have then been included with each scenario. You may well think of other points in addition to these. The notes accompanying each scenario are by no means complete but may stimulate further discussion. More practice questions may be found in Chapter 6.

SCENARIO 1: INTRODUCING A NEW SERVICE IN THE PRACTICE

You are a GP registrar, have recently completed a minor surgical course and are keen to perform surgical procedures in your practice. A meeting is held with the senior partner, lead nurse and practice manager [other candidates]. Your role is to persuade the other members of the team that it is a good idea.

(If you have the chance to practise this scenario in a group, each of you may want to introduce a service to the surgery and the team should debate which service is best. Other services may include an obesity clinic, an echocardiography service or a breast-feeding clinic.)

NOTES

- Can you demonstrate the need for the service by reviewing the number of surgical referrals to secondary care and by patient feedback? (Audit)
- What procedures can you perform?
- It can offer your patients a fast and local service.
- What happens if things go wrong?
- What extra equipment do you need?
- Who will see your usual GP patients while you are operating? Will you need locum cover?
- What quality assurance can you offer?
- Do you need on-going training?
- Will you need an assistant? If that assistant is your practice nurse, will she be taken out of her usual clinics?
- Is it financially viable for the practice? Will you be able to offer it as a service to the local practices? Will the primary care trust (PCT) reimburse you because you are saving them money? You will need to formulate a business plan.
- When do you plan on implementing the service?

SCENARIO 2: ALLOCATION OF FUNDS

The practice had received a donation of £2000 from a local charity. Four GP partners attend a meeting, of which you are one, to discuss how to spend the money. Two of you would like to buy an ambulatory blood pressure monitor (ABPM) for the practice whereas the other two GPs would like to decorate the reception area which has become quite shabby. What are the issues? Can you reach an agreement?

NOTES

- £2000 is a lot of money. Was it donated legitimately without bribe or obligation? The General Medical Council (GMC) has published guidelines on the receipt of gifts.
- Patients with borderline or presumptive white coat hypertension often require a number of separate clinic appointments to measure blood pressure. Labelling them as hypertensive and treating patients with medication may have a number of implications, including psychological and financial, eg health insurance. An ABPM can help confirm the presence or absence of hypertension, save on clinic appointments and save having to refer borderline patients to secondary care for ambulatory monitoring. There is much pressure to reduce referral activity to secondary care. Who will administer the ABPM and analyse the results? Will it need servicing and calibration? Will the nurses need training to fit the monitor?
- The reception area should be inviting, comfortable, safe for staff and patients, and offer confidentiality when patients are discussing their business at reception. With the new GMS contract, more patients provide more income to the practice. An attractive reception area gives a professional and organised image to the practice. Prospective patients may find this inviting. Does the current reception area offer these qualities?
- Did last year's patient survey contain any comments about the reception area? Practices are paid under the new contract to undertake a standardised satisfaction survey.
- Can a proportion of the money be spent on reception and a smaller amount on another piece of equipment?
- Respect for each other's views is important.
- Keep an open mind. Consider what is important, ie the practice and patients, not personal gains.
- Aggressive dictatorial styles will not be rewarded; the examiners want to see team players, the ability to see all points of view, negotiation, and willingness to lead and compromise when appropriate.

SCENARIO 3: SETTING UP A SERVICE IN THE LOCAL AREA

You are the cardiology lead in the practice and feel the need to set up a specialist clinic in the local area, focusing on primary prevention for cardiovascular disease. Your practice colleagues are on board and a meeting has been set up. Other attendees include a GP from another practice, the prescribing lead for the PCT and the PCT commissioning lead. What are the issues?

NOTES

- Ischaemic heart disease is the number one killer in the UK: screening could be directed at high-risk groups only.
- What are the benefits?
  - primary prevention can reduce the pressure on secondary care, making better use of resources
  - public health should improve
  - screening may uncover previously undiagnosed hypertension, diabetes, hypercholesterolaemia
  - smoking cessation clinics have many health benefits.
- What are the risks/downsides?
  - financial implications
  - Will other practices lose out on possible financial gain?
  - patients will require regular follow-up to maintain lifestyle change
  - the clinics will take health staff away from routine clinics in an already struggling NHS
  - Where will the patients be seen? How will patients access the service if they live far away?
  - may upset local GPs – their workload may increase, eg patients with newly diagnosed diabetes.
- Resources:
  - financial
  - premises
  - clinical staff
  - secretarial support
  - phlebotomy
  - IT
  - communications.
- Audit:
  - quality assurance required
    - regular audit:
    - how frequently?
    - what is audited
    - who oversees the audit?
    - probity.

SCENARIO 4: DEALING WITH A COMPLAINT

A number of patients have made complaints against a receptionist. She has been at the practice for 23 years and is loved by all the doctors. The doctors and practice manager hold a meeting to discuss the complaints. Each of you has a separate complaint to present to the meeting. What issues does this situation raise? What should the team do next?

Complaints

- A patient was refused an emergency appointment

- A prescription was lost

- Failure to answer the telephones quickly

- Poor personal hygiene.

NOTES

- To whom were the complaints made? Were the complaints put in writing to the practice manager or merely comments at the front desk? If they were comments to other members of staff, were they true or hearsay?
- There needs to be an investigation and, if an official complaint has been made by a patient, it should be acknowledged in writing within 2 working days and an appropriate response in 10 days.
- What is the gravity of the complaint? What are the consequences?
- Is the offence disciplinary? Consider discussing with a medical defence union or employment adviser. If the offence is severe enough to require a disciplinary, a strict procedure must be followed.
- The receptionist may require performance management.
- Are there systems within the practice that led to the problem?
- Was she under stress? Why?
- Is she depressed or does she have a physical problem? Should she see her own GP?
- A meeting will need to be held with the member of staff. Her version of events will be required. Who will lead that meeting? How will it affect her long-term relationship with the practice?

SCENARIO 5: ADVERTISING IN THE SURGERY

A patient, whom you have known for many years, has come to see you, a GP partner, in surgery asking if she can leave some leaflets in the waiting room. The leaflets promote her new weight loss business. The diet is a low-calorie formula that she developed with her sister. You suggest to the patient that you will discuss the issue at a practice meeting. The other attendees of the meeting include the practice manager and diabetes nurse.

NOTES

- How does it make you feel as her doctor?
- Is she abusing the doctor–patient relationship and her relationship with the practice or is she innocently asking for a favour? How will the relationship be affected if the decision is no?
- What is the science behind the diet? Is there any evidence supporting its use and safety?
- Weight loss is a major issue nationally. Diabetes is one of the many sequelae. Should patients be offered as much help as possible?
- The quality outcomes framework (QOF; see p92) points may be improved if patients lose weight, with lower blood pressure and better diabetes control for example. In that case shouldn't they be offered it on the NHS?
- If the practice allows leaflets to be left in the waiting room, are they condoning the diet? What happens if another patient then suffers ill health as a result of going on the diet? Will the practice be implicated? Should the leaflets have a disclaimer?
- Will patients assume that the surgery is making a profit?
- It is best to say to the patient that it will have to be discussed at a meeting. A letter outlining the final decision should be signed by all partners or the practice manager to limit damaging the relationship between the patient and her doctor.

SCENARIO 6: EMPLOYING MORE STAFF

One of the practice doctors said that the practice
population has increased recently and suggested that you
need more clinical staff to cope with the pressure. What
are the issues? Four GP partners attend the meeting.

NOTES

- Has there been a genuine increase in practice population? Most GP computer systems should provide these data. Consultation rates for each doctor and nurse should be reviewed.
- If there has not been an increase in total demand, why is it that the individual perceives a greater workload? Has he been put upon? Do other members of staff feel like this? Is there more paperwork or home visits than last year? Is that member of staff pressured for other reasons – managerial jobs or stress at home perhaps? Does the workload need to be shared more equally?
- If there has been an increase, can the extra workload be dealt with more efficiently rather than employing more staff? Do nurses have spaces in their clinic? Could they see minor illness patients? Could a health-care assistant (HCA) be employed for phlebotomy, ECGs and spirometry? The nurses could therefore see more minor illness and chronic disease, freeing up the doctors to manage more complicated problems? What are the nurses' views? This may be more cost-effective.
- Is there enough physical space to have an HCA as well as nurses?
- Is it cheaper to pay another practice for their services or to rent a room from them?
- Should the practice close their lists?
- Do some doctors offer too many follow-ups or order too many investigations, eg bloods and ECGs, that drain practice resources unnecessarily?

SCENARIO 7: PRIVATE SCREENING

A local screening company has approached you wanting
to screen your practice population for osteoporosis.
Patients will be charged for the service. They have offered
your practice a financial incentive and support staff. What
are the issues? A GP partner, practice nurse and practice
manager attend the meeting.

NOTES

- There has been recent negative publicity on this issue, with possible legal action against the practices concerned.
- The service may generate income to the practice.
- What is the evidence for screening? Is there a health benefit? If there is, should GPs be making money on it or should they be offering the service for free? Hip fractures have a significant mortality and there are treatments available for osteoporosis.
- What image does it promote for the practice?
- Consider discussing the offer with local medical committee (LMC), a medical defence union or the PCT.
- How do the local orthopaedic/rheumatology consultants feel about it?
- Should the practice divulge patient information to a third party? Is this unlawful?
- What are the probity issues here?
- Would it be acceptable if the money were invested back into patient care?

SCENARIO 8: THE LOCAL COMMUNITY

A local parents' committee want you to sign a
petition against a local firm; they plan to erect a
telecommunication pole in the village. Four partners from
the practice meet to discuss the situation. What are the
issues?

NOTES

- Who is it on the parents' committee that wants you to sign the petition? Do you know their background? Do they have issues themselves?
- What is the concern about the pole? Is it a medical concern or is there another agenda, eg defacing the village? Is there any medical evidence that the telecom pole is a risk to public health?
- How do the other partners feel about it? Is your signing or not signing it a reflection of the practice's view?
- The press may comment on doctors signing or not signing the petition. How will that affect the practice's reputation in the village? Could the practice lose patients? Income depends on the number of patients registered with the practice under the new GP GMS contract.
- How will the firm feel about it? Are their employees registered with the practice? Does the practice perform private medicals on the firm's employees that generate income? If there is medical evidence against the pole, is it unethical not to sign the petition in case the practice loses the medical contract?
- What are the advantages to the local community in having a telecom pole? For example, better mobile phone coverage.
- Is there a view from the public health team?
- Are there other issues that you can think of?

SCENARIO 9: DEALING WITH PROBLEM COLLEAGUES

You suspect that Dr A Buse, one of your colleagues, has been abusing alcohol. Another of your colleagues attending the meeting has also smelt alcohol on Dr Buse's breath. Four of the doctors attend a meeting to discuss how to manage the situation.

NOTES

- Dealing with colleagues is a common theme in general practice assessments. Doctors may face significant pressures for a number of different reasons. Pressure may affect the doctor's medical performance and affect behaviour. Behaviours of concern include alcohol or drug abuse, inappropriate behaviour towards patients, stealing, self-prescribing antidepressants, etc.

- The GMC offer guidance on this; it is imperative that you are familiar with this. There are a huge number of issues on this subject:

  What is the problem?

  How did the problem present itself?

  Who was affected and how? How has it affected the practice?

  Is there a safety issue that needs addressing immediately, was there medical mismanagement?

  Should the GP's consultations be checked?

  Has there been a criminal offence?

  Why did the issue happen?

  Has the GP been under pressure from the workplace?

  Are there pressures at home?

  Is there drug or alcohol misuse?

  Is there mental illness?

  Should the GP be suspended or does he need support? Does he need time off?

  Should the doctor be performance managed?

Chapter 4
Prioritisation Exercises

PRIORITISATION EXERCISES

The very nature of medicine requires doctors to deal with a number of tasks throughout the working day. When faced with a series of jobs, doctors must prioritise the order in which they should be dealt with. The prioritisation exercise is a written assessment designed to test a number of different skills under the national person specification (NPS).

Around five tasks are presented and the candidate is required to rank the order in which they should be dealt with. Some deaneries will require the candidate to put a series of tasks in order of priority, eg A–E, whereas others may expect a written paragraph justifying the answer. There is no right or wrong answer to this section of the assessment as long as sensible reasoning is offered. Candidates have approximately 30 minutes to write their answers although there may be variations between deaneries. Clear writing (perhaps using bullet points), and logical and clear arguments demonstrate clear thinking. Scribbles and crossings out will not inspire the assessors.

Clinical knowledge and expertise are required to prioritise safely. The consequences of delaying care should be considered when faced with a number of tasks. The complexity of some tasks may not always be apparent, eg the duty (on-call) doctor may be required to call a patient back because he or she has 'run out of their pills'. Of course, it may be that the patient has a long-standing chronic illness and merely requires more of his or her drugs. On the other hand, the patient may be experiencing chest pain, but rather than 'bothering the doctor' he or she has called the surgery and asked for more GTN spray. Hence, conceptual thinking and problem-solving skills are tested.

Although general practices tend to be supportive and enjoyable environments in which to work, there may be times when the duty day gets busy. Stress develops when you feel overwhelmed by the number or nature of tasks at hand. Once pressure exceeds a certain point, anxiety increases, causing mental ability and performance to fall. The consequences can be disastrous. A GP must be able to cope with pressure when managing multiple tasks but, at the same time, recognise when help is required and be able to look after him- or herself. Robust organisational skills and appropriate delegation to doctor colleagues or other members of staff may be required when managing a series of tasks; these are mentioned in the NPS.

There are some guiding principles that may be used when prioritising tasks:

- There is often more than one way to manage a series of tasks.
- Consider splitting the tasks into urgent and non-urgent. Then prioritise each of these groups in turn.
- Can you justify your actions?
- Safety is paramount.
- Never cut corners.
- Can you delegate any tasks?
- Let your colleagues know that you are under pressure. Can they help? Use the team.
- Make sure that you manage your stress appropriately.
- Do not automatically put personal issues last. Failure to deal with a personal crisis may affect your concentration.
- Do not risk your own physical or mental health.
- What can you do differently next time?

CHAPTER 4

' I speak from bitter experience when I recommend that you take a watch with you if only for the written section, as this can be tight for time if you want to say all the things that you think will help you stand out from the crowd. We had about half an hour to answer questions relating to a scenario in which we were a busy junior doctor being asked to prioritise a number of jobs. I tried to demonstrate that I can tackle a problem by making a clear plan, that I can practise safe medicine, and that I am a team player who can both delegate and humbly seek help. With this scenario I felt it important to emphasise the need to be working as part of a team that was communicating, and constantly reviewing changes as they happened ... . '

Dr Duncan Rourke

Stage 2 GP VTS

CHAPTER 4

PRACTICE SCENARIOS

It may be helpful to work though the following questions on your own, and then discuss the answers with your colleagues. There are no right or wrong answers, as long as you can justify your actions. Suggested answers have been given. Spaces have been provided for your answers and the thought processes behind them.

SCENARIO 1: DUTY DOCTOR – F1 (MEDICAL)

You're an F1 doctor on call. There are five more patients to see. Put the following in the most appropriate order, justifying your answer:

A   Clerk Miss Smith who has been referred by her GP with a week's history of lower limb cellulitis. Her vitals are stable.

B   See Mr Patel who has been referred by accident and emergency for pleuritic chest pain. He has already been given low-molecular-weight heparin and is awaiting the result of the D-dimer blood test. He is not breathless and is comfortable. The A&E nurses are keeping an eye on him.

C   Attend Mrs Ayoola who has been having palpitations.

D   Treat Mr Stevens, aged 27, with type 1 diabetes. His blood sugars have climbed to 26 mmol/L today. His saw his GP yesterday morning for a urinary tract infection and was given antibiotics.

E   Miss Morris needs her discharge letter and has been waiting all day. She is angry.

CHAPTER 4

NOTES

Suggested answer: C D E A B

This question tests a number of criteria within the NPS including: organisation and planning; conceptual thinking and problem-solving; coping with pressure; empathy and sensitivity; clinical knowledge and expertise.

Mrs Ayoola is in hospital with palpitations. She should be reviewed first; after all, there is little information about the nature of palpitations, whether she has associated chest pain, breathlessness or dizziness, or any co-morbidities. You should establish whether her symptoms are the result of a benign or malignant cardiac rhythm and treat accordingly.

Mr Stevens' diabetic control has deteriorated. You must establish whether he is in diabetic ketoacidosis (DKA) and also why his blood sugars have gone up. It is likely that the urinary tract infection is to blame, although you must consider non-infective causes such as poor drug compliance and myocardial infarction. Failure to treat the DKA may prove fatal.

Miss Morris is understandably angry for having to wait and her discharge paperwork should be done as soon as it is safe to do so. An apology, briefly explaining why you were delayed, may help her understand why she had to wait. Her letter should only take a few moments. Although cellulitis can cause sepsis, Miss Smith is stable. Mr Patel is already on treatment for a possible pulmonary embolus and he is being monitored in A&E.

CHAPTER 4

SCENARIO 2: DUTY DOCTOR – GP

You are the duty doctor at your GP practice and have just finished a busy clinic when the receptionist calls – a patient with severe abdominal pain has just walked into the waiting room. The practice manager then walks into your room; she is in tears over the terrible way the government have treated GPs. You then receive a text message on your mobile phone, to call your child-minder urgently. Jenny, the prescriptions clerk starts to talk over you and the manager, demanding that the prescriptions are signed immediately, the pharmacist is waiting to pick them up. How do you manage the situation?

NOTES

- Safety is paramount. If you do not call your child-minder first, you may not be able to concentrate properly. Your child may be seriously unwell. It is not unreasonable briefly to call your child-minder and establish what is going on. If you have to act quickly you may have to ask another colleague to see the patient in the waiting room.

- The patient in the waiting room may have a sinister cause for the abdominal pain and ought to be triaged as soon as possible. Abdominal pain may have a sinister cause.

- Although the practice manager is upset, it is best to explain that you cannot really talk about government policy right now. Mentioning that you cannot talk because of an unwell patient will stop her feeling undervalued.

- Although the prescriptions have to be signed at some point, they do not have to be signed immediately. A quick apology to the pharmacist will go a long way. Perhaps, once they are signed, they could be dropped off to the chemist by another member of staff. Can someone else sign the prescriptions?

- The two most important issues here are the patient with the abdominal pain and checking out what the issue is with the child-minder. It is important to keep your cool, maintain your manners and try to delegate if possible. If you do lose your cool with staff, an apology goes a long way; they may have felt under pressure too.

CHAPTER 4

SCENARIO 3: DUTY DOCTOR – F1 (SURGICAL)

You are a surgical F1 doctor on call for the wards and accident and emergency. Your registrar and consultant have been delayed in theatre. There are a number of patients waiting for your attention. Whom do you see first and why?

A   Miss Gardiner has been referred by the accident and emergency department (A&E) with a diagnosis of appendicitis. Her pregnancy test is negative. She is stable.

B   Mr Singh, a postoperative patient, has suddenly become breathless and tachycardic.

C   Mr Rahman's catheter has blocked again and needs changing. He is feeling a little uncomfortable

D   Mr Ford has been complaining of a painful red calf after his recent operation. He is otherwise well.

E   Mrs Cartwright has been complaining of pain around her cannula site. It has become red and painful. She is well in herself.

NOTES

Suggested answer: B A D C E

- Mr Singh needs urgent attention. There are a number of differential diagnoses including a pulmonary embolus, acute left ventricular failure, hypovolaemia, myocardial infarction and drug reaction.

- Leaving a patient with appendicitis could be dangerous, the appendix could burst and the patient may be left in pain. Given that the A&E doctor has already seen the patient, perhaps you may ask your registrar to review the patient. If your registrar is busy, you should review Miss Gardiner once Mr Singh has been stabilised.

- Mr Ford may have a deep vein thrombosis. He is well but should be seen next so that the diagnosis can be confirmed and treatment commenced. There is a risk of embolic disease.

- Mr Rahman's catheter is blocked and not for the first time. While he is in a little discomfort, his condition is not immediately life threatening. Can the ward sister or night nurse change the catheter?

- Mrs Cartwright has a likely infection secondary to intravenous access. She will need to have the cannula taken out and sited elsewhere as well as antibiotics. It is highly unlikely that she will deteriorate before you treat the other patients.

SCENARIO 4: DUTY DOCTOR – GP

You are the duty doctor in your practice. Your colleagues are in a meeting and are unavailable. The list of duty jobs is as follows:

A   Mr Morris, diarrhoea, 3 days, getting worse, wants home visit.

B   Please call Dr Hendry at Queen's Hospital, bleep 2866, re your referral on Mrs Aitcheson last week.

C   Please call Sarah Smith, wants advice, did not say why.

D   Please call Steven Lord, going on holiday tonight, needs to see you a.s.a.p. re asthma.

E   Juliette [your practice manager] wants a word; please call her after surgery.

F   Harold Knight, chest pain – at King George nursing home.

Put the jobs in order of priority, justifying your answer.

NOTES

Suggested answer: D F C A E B

- Steven Lord could well need some asthma inhalers in which case it will take 2 minutes to call and find out. An alternative scenario, however, could be that he is struggling to breathe and is desperate for his inhalers. In this case you can arrange treatment straight away. The receptionists will put their own interpretation of the patient's complaint on the job list and it is the duty doctor's responsibility to ensure that the patient is ok. Asthma still kills around 1500 patients per year in the UK.

- Harold Knight may have a sinister cause for his pain. When did the call come through? This could be triaged over the phone in the first instance. It may be that it is a clear case for an emergency ambulance. He is in a nursing home where health-care professionals can monitor him closely until he receives further care. An ambulance may be inappropriate; perhaps he has an advanced directive. This being the case, you will have to visit the patient as soon as possible. Should the receptionists have called you out of surgery for a patient with chest pain? Do they know to call you out of surgery for chest pain and other significant symptoms? Consider holding a significant event analysis.

- Sarah Smith should be called next. Her reason for calling needs to be ascertained and prioritised. It may be that she wants her chlamydia results; perhaps she is worried about her husband's COPD or maybe has 'indigestion', which is actually pain originating from a cardiac source. You could ask the receptionist to gather more information; however, the issue may be sensitive, a rape, for example.

- Mr Morris's diarrhoea may be managed over the phone if he is well in himself. In certain circumstances, in addition to asking him if his mouth is wet or dry, you may be able to ask him to assess his capillary refill time and pulse. If there are no concerning features, discussion of oral rehydration therapy and safety netting is appropriate. Even though patients want home visits, quite often they can come into the practice or may be managed with telephone advice.

- A quick call to your practice manager may be the next job on the list. A quick apology for any delay would be appropriate. It could be that she knows that you have been busy and asked if you would like some lunch or perhaps a more pressing issue within the practice. Can the issue wait? Can it be delegated to any of the other doctors within the practice?

- Dr Hendry should be contacted, apologising for the delay, when you have time. It is worth looking at the record. Did you or a colleague refer Mrs Aitcheson? If it was not you, ask the referring GP to make the call (assuming that the GP is working today). Dr Hendry may think that the referral is inappropriate, that it may better dealt with by another speciality; perhaps he needs more information or would like some preliminary tests performed before she comes to the clinic.

CHAPTER 4

Chapter 5
Important Topics

CHAPTER 5

IMPORTANT TOPICS

These topics may come up during various parts of the stage 3 assessment. Although an understanding of the topics is required rather than a detailed knowledge, their application will impress the assessors.

MULTIDISCIPLINARY TEAM

An appreciation of the practice and multidisciplinary team may be demonstrated in all the exercises within stage 3:

- The community team:
  - general practice receptionists: take phone calls, book appointments
  - admin staff: note summarising, repeat prescription management, management of hospital letters – scanning them into notes, buildings maintenance, rotas, patient recall for chronic disease clinics and immunisations
  - secretaries: patient liaison, dealing with correspondence and dictation, communication with outside agencies
  - financial manager, practice manager
  - health-care assistants: take blood, ECGs, spirometry, wound care, blood pressure checks
  - nurses
  - specialist nurses, eg diabetes
  - counsellor
  - salaried GP, GP partners (own the practice)
  - community staff: include specialist cancer nurses, community heart failure nurses, district nurses.

ETHICAL DILEMMAS

- GPs may face ethical dilemmas on a daily basis. Without a framework to help make these sometimes complex decisions, you may find it impossible reach a conclusion. A number of texts have been published to help understand the basic ethical principles and medical law. Reading through these guides may put you at a significant advantage during your career as a GP. A basic ethical framework to use is as follows:
  - *autonomy* – respecting the patient's wishes. Normally this trumps the other concepts described here; there will be circumstances, however, where this is not always the case
  - *beneficence* – to do good
  - *non-maleficence* – to do no harm
  - *justice* – in the public interest.

Consider the following example:

Mr Harold Smith is an 80-year-old man with dementia. He has lived with his wife, Margaret, in the same house since they were married 61 years ago. Except for arthritis, she is well. She needs twice-weekly hydrotherapy to help with her joint pains. Mr Smith drives her to her sessions. He loves driving and feels that it gives him independence. Last week, he reversed into a lamppost and the previous week, he nearly hit a child. Using an ethical framework, how do you manage the situation?

Mr Smith would clearly love to continue driving; taking that privilege away from him can have disastrous consequences for both him and his wife. Although autonomy normal trumps the other ethical arguments above, it does not in this case. It may do harm to the couple to suggest that he should not drive anymore; however, the consequences of a car accident are a lot greater. Justice, for the good of the public, therefore dictates that he should not drive. Transport can be arranged for Mrs Smith and charities may help with local trips.

SIGNIFICANT EVENT ANALYSIS

Significant event analysis may well come up in stage 3 during the group discussion or the interview. It may also be known as critical event analysis. A critical/significant event is an adverse event that occurs in the workplace. The incident may not necessarily be a clinical issue although it often is. A patient complaint or a serious diagnosis, eg cancer, could be considered. A significant event analysis is then carried out and discussed to tease out what happened, and work out the chain of events that led to the adverse outcome. How did it affect the patient, the staff and the practice/hospital? Could any systems be introduced or modified to ensure that it does not happen again? What audits are required? An example of a critical event form is given below.

Significant event analysis

(presented by *name*)

Date:

What happened?

How did it affect:

Me?

Patient?

Practice?

Could it have been avoided?

How can it be prevented from happening again?

Learning needs

CHAPTER 5

AUDIT

This is a clinical governance tool designed to appraise your practice and is relevant to the group discussion as well as the interview. All doctors should look at their own work and the work of their department, to assess whether they are treating their patient population to an appropriate standard. Of course, many doctors may think that they are treating their patients to a high standard. Audit helps to prove, or disprove, that assumption. Audit is likely to be part of revalidation. Take the following scenario:

> It may be that all the doctors in a practice think that they monitor renal function after introducing ACE (angiotensin-converting enzyme) inhibitors. Perhaps an educational course or even a critical event brought it to the attention of one of the doctors that maybe they don't always check renal function appropriately. The doctor could hide the issue from the rest of the team and merely change his or her own practice. Hiding the incident brings into question the doctor's professional integrity. The doctor could audit all patients started on ACE inhibitors within the practice to review how many patients do actually have their bloods checked. The vast majority of general practices are computerised, so it would be easy to search for the data. In hospital, the process of getting the paper notes can be arduous.

The criterion could be that renal function should be checked within 2 weeks of starting ACE inhibitors. The audit standard could be that 90 per cent of patients should have their bloods checked within 2 weeks of drug commencement. Why not 100 per cent? Often logistical reasons mean that achieving 100 per cent is unrealistic, eg patients or staff being on holiday.

An initial notes review is performed to assess how the practice is currently performing. If the number of patients having their renal function checked is actually below what is acceptable, the practice can introduce a system to ensure that the audit standard is achieved. Once the new system is in place, another review can be performed to see if the intervention has been successful. Subsequent searches should be carried out to ensure that the practice maintains the audit standard.

AUDIT CYCLE

1. Identify need for audit (new guideline, adverse clinical event, reflective practice)
2. What is the criterion? What are you actually auditing?
3. Set audit standard
4. Initial data collection: has your standard been reached?
5. Introduce change/system to improve your standard
6. Secondary data collection: has your standard improved? If not, why not? If so, can you improve it any more?
7. Regular data collection to ensure that standard is maintained.

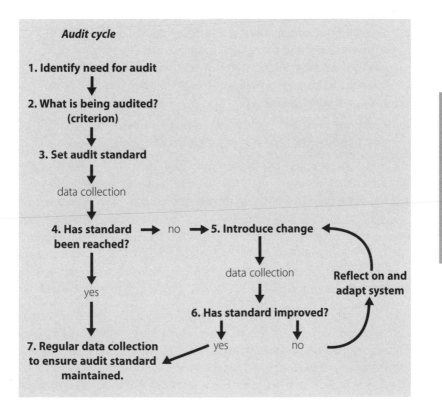

Audit cycle

1. Identify need for audit
↓
2. What is being audited? (criterion)
↓
3. Set audit standard
↓
data collection
↓
4. Has standard been reached? → no → **5. Introduce change** ←
↓ yes | data collection | **Reflect on and adapt system**
| ↓
| **6. Has standard improved?**
7. Regular data collection to ensure audit standard maintained. ← yes | no

THE CYCLE OF CHANGE

The cycle of change was developed by psychologists Prochaska and DiClemente (1983). It may be applied to any patient when managing a change in behaviour and is likely to be relevant in the mock consultation. Take smoking: a patient who already smokes may thoroughly enjoy it, may be thinking about giving up or perhaps has planned a quit programme. This being the case, if a patient who is already keen to give up receives a lecture from a GP on the dangers of smoking, he or she may be frustrated with the care that he or she receives from the GP. The GP may feel that he or she has done his or her job but, in reality, has failed. Ascertaining what the patient's views are on smoking is a good way of gauging where he or she is in the cycle of change. That way, the patient can be helped and will feel listened to. The following are the stages in the process of change:

1. Precontemplation: patient enjoying behaviour, little motivation to change – eating too much, smoking, etc. Doctor's role is to get the patient thinking that it would be in the patient's health interests to change behaviour. This may move the patient on to the contemplation stage.

2. Contemplation: patient is thinking that he or she should give up the behaviour but has not planned how to go about it.

3. Preparation: active management plan to give up the behaviour, eg smoking counselling, start nicotine replacement, phased reduction in number of cigarettes smoked.

4. Action: quit date.

5. Maintenance: period of time that patient abstains from behaviour.

6. Relapse: patient resumes behaviour, but may try to quit again in the future.

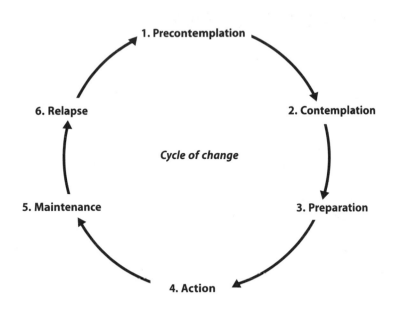

Adapted from Prochaska and Diclemente (1983)

MANAGEMENT OF CHANGE

Some parts of the stage 3 examination, particularly the team exercise, may require a candidate to present an idea to the rest of the practice team (the other candidates) and persuade them that the idea is a sound one. The idea will invariably involve a change in the way that the practice operates or a change in behaviour from the staff. Introducing a change is not always easy and may require extra effort from the practice team, time and money. As such, the science of management of change has evolved. Without a leader who is passionate about their idea, it will not become a reality. What the idea is, why it is important, the risks and benefits to the practice, the implications, what is required from whom, the resources required, timescale, implementation and audit plans must be presented to all those who may be affected (stakeholders).

THE NEW GENERAL MEDICAL SERVICES CONTRACT

General practitioners voted on a new contract that came into effect in 2004. The contract is between the practice and the primary care trust (PCT) rather than individual GPs. A cursory knowledge of the new General Medical Services (nGMS) contract may be particularly relevant to the group exercise, if a debate about practice funding arises for example.

The income from the nGMS contract follows the patient; in other words, the more patients on the practice list, the more money the practice can generate. Funding follows a number of different streams:
*   Global sum – to cover the provision of both essential and additional services
*   Enhanced services
*   Quality outcomes framework.

There are five different types of service.

ESSENTIAL SERVICES

These are mandatory and cover provision of health care to anyone who is sick or 'believes themselves to be sick', including emergency care and care for patients with chronic diseases.

Practices can either opt in or out of the following services, depending on staffing issues, training, etc. Also, if a practice feels that they are not being paid enough to provide a particular service, they could decide not to provide it.

ADDITIONAL SERVICES

This comprises services such as child health surveillance, contraception, cervical screening, childhood immunisations, and antenatal and postnatal care, ie services that most GPs routinely provide at present.

DIRECTED ENHANCED SERVICES (DES)

These services are more specialised. The primary care organisation (PCO) is expected to ensure provision of these services somehow, but not all practices will offer everything. Examples are care of violent patients and minor surgery (not cryotherapy and curettage, which are 'additional services').

NATIONAL ENHANCED SERVICES (NES)

The PCO itself will decide whether to provide these services, eg a rural PCO might decide not to provide additional services for the homeless. Examples of NESs include drug misuse services, care for homeless people, fitting an intrauterine contraceptive device (IUCD), anticoagulant services, intrapartum care and minor injury services.

LOCAL ENHANCED SERVICES (LES)

These services are tailored to local needs, eg care of refugees.

QUALITY OUTCOMES FRAMEWORK

The quality outcomes framework (QOF) provides an additional funding stream to practice. Around a third of practice income is generated through the QOF. A number of points are achievable through various different domains, both clinical and non-clinical. The disease prevalence of each condition can affect how valuable each point is. Complex software is used to monitor how well each practice is doing and to calculate the final achievement.

QUALITY DOMAINS

- Clinical: cardiovascular disease (CVD), heart failure, stroke, diabetes, hypertension, COPD, asthma, mental health, depression, learning disabilities, epilepsy, thyroid disease, cancer, dementia, chronic kidney disease, obesity, smoking.
- Organisational: records, information, communication, education and training, practice management and medicines management.
- Patient experience: validated questionnaires should be used.
- Additional services: cervical screening, child health surveillance, maternity services, contraception.
- Holistic: for achievement across the whole clinical area.

(See Department of Health website, www.dh.gov.uk)

OTHER IMPORTANT POINTS IN THE NEW CONTRACT

- Most GPs 'opted out' of 24-hour responsibility at a cost of 6 per cent of the global sum, which is approximately £6000/GP per year.
- Seniority payments start earlier and increase year by year. They are based on the date of GMC registration, not the number of years worked as a GP. However, controversially, they are linked to the profitability of the practice, so low-earning principals (eg part-time partners) will be penalised.
- Information technology, eg computers bought and owned by PCT.

PERSONAL MEDICAL SERVICES

Some practices have a personal medical services (PMS) contract rather than an nGMS one. PMS contracts are negotiated locally between the practice and the PCT and are truly tailored to the needs of the local population. The nGMS is a nationally negotiated contract.

CHAPTER 5

PRIMARY CARE TRUST

An understanding of the structure of the PCT is essential for GPs and is relevant, in particular, to the team exercise. General practices have a contract with their local PCT and are in constant communication with them. The PCT is responsible for the provision and budgeting of health care for both primary (community) and secondary (hospital) medicine.

- Free-standing statutory bodies
- Provide primary and community services
- Coordinate, manage and provide funding
- Commissioners of care, although much commissioning under practice-based commissioning (PBC)
- Responsibilities:
  - to provide health services to local people
  - to administer the budget
  - to be publicly accountable
  - to employ and manage community staff
  - to fund independent contractors in health care – including dentists, optometrists and pharmacists
  - to maintain and improve quality
  - to implement poor performance procedures
  - to encourage evidence-based practice
  - to monitor services
  - answers to strategic health authority, local people, Healthcare Commission, government
- People:
  - board with chair
  - CEO (chief executive officer)
  - PEC (professional executive committee) – leads and guides the PCT
  - senior management
  - clinical leads
  - educational leads – nurse/GP tutor
  - prescribing leads – usually a manager/pharmacist and a GP.

OUT OF HOURS

As part of the new GP contract, GPs opted out of out-of-hours (OOH) responsibility. In other words, most GP practices will be responsible for the provision of care to their patients between 8am and 6.30pm. This costs GPs approximately £6000/year, which does not cover the cost of providing the service. Despite the nGMS contact and OOH provision being agreed, there is increasing pressure from government for GPs to work more unsociable hours. This may be relevant, particularly in the group exercise when discussing the way in which the practice operates.

- PCT responsibility to provide OOH care – commonly through a private provider company.
- Many models, eg
  - GPs and nurses triage calls and see patients at base or at home
  - paramedics see patients at home and bring patient to base if doctor required
  - all patients receive home visits.
- Recent Department of Health (DH) intervention when a PCT set up a doctor-free OOH service.
- Some areas already having problems covering shifts.
- Implications for training GPs.
- Issues for patients: less continuity of care, OOH services have no access to patient records, patients have to travel further to see an on-call doctor, longer waiting times before patient can receive health care.
- Issues for doctors: better quality of life, opportunity to work for the OOH service, new career option, de-skilled in emergency general practice, increased daytime workload?

CHAPTER 5

CHOOSE AND BOOK

Choose and book may be relevant during the mock consultation when explaining the referral process to patients. It may also be relevant to the group discussion.

- Introduced in 2006.
- It allows patients to choose which secondary care centre their GP refers them to. Patient then calls to make an appointment that suits them.
- GPs counsel patients on which services are available – list of services provided online.
- Online system provides information to GPs and patients including transport links and waiting times.
- Patients require a password and reference number, provided by GP, before appointment can be made.
- GP then sends electronic referral letter to patient's chosen hospital.
- Empowers patients, allows doctors to track referrals, quick electronic referrals, should reduce non-attendance as patients choose an appointment that suits them.
- Who takes responsibility if patients do not call to arrange appointment? Illiterate patients may be disadvantaged. Choose and book is heavily dependent on technology, which is costly to install. The process is time-consuming for GPs in an already time-pressured environment. Some patient information is uploaded onto the NHS Spine – how secure is this?

PRACTICE-BASED COMMISSIONING (PBC)

Services in the community may be offered at a cheaper tariff than the hospital can provide. Under PBC, GP practices can commission or provide services for their patients. Groups of practices across the country have formed 'collaboratives' that commission services. GPs and private companies can also provide and deliver services to the local area, eg vasectomies, and generate income. PBC may be discussed in the group exercise, particularly when debating new practice services or generating income:

- Target was to have all practices involved by end of 2006.
- PCT will bear the risk.
- Proportion of savings will be used for patient care (eg new equipment).
- Drivers: payment by results and increasing hospital costs, savings for practices, more control of services provided.
- Increased patient choice.

CHAPTER 5

APPRAISAL AND REVALIDATION

- Appraisal is a formative and developmental process – for the benefit of the appraisee.
- Based around the headings in Good Medical Practice (GMC).
- Annual appraisal was voluntary – can take independent route to revalidation, but has become a contractual requirement
- NHS Appraisal Toolkit: background preparation for appraisal completed online.
- Appraisal divided into subheadings:
  - good clinical care
  - maintaining good medical practice
  - relationships with patients
  - working with colleagues
  - teaching and training
  - probity
  - management activity
  - research
  - health.
- Appraisal summary sent to a lead clinician at the PCT, who should collate educational needs information for the PCT, so that they can provide a targeted education programme.
- The PCT is responsible for the process.
- Evidence that poorly performing doctors do not look after their educational and developmental needs, and that those who do perform better.
- Every doctor will be required to be revalidated every 5 years.
- Think about:
  - formative vs summative
  - whether the system will find poor performers
  - will it be threatening?
  - issues around confidentiality/honesty, etc
  - takes time to prepare and to do
  - benefits and risks.

NATIONAL CLINICAL ASSESSMENT SERVICE (NCAS)

- Organisation that offers advice and assessment of poorly performing doctors to PCTs.
- New guidance on poor performance management advises involving them at early stage.
- It is concerned with looking at doctors and dentists for whom fitness to practise is in doubt but not certain.
- Liaises closely with the GMC when indicated.
- Panel of trained assessors – in each speciality.
- Assessment team: manager, two doctors (one or both same speciality as doctor being assessed) and lay person.
- Reports advice on remedial action: usually about education and support – the PCT has to provide or facilitate this, often with local deanery.

NATIONAL INSTITUTE FOR HEALTH AND CLINICAL EXCELLENCE (NICE)

Some group exercises or mock consultations may involve discussion about drugs, eg patients may request expensive drugs not approved by NICE or the PCT prescribing team.

- Delivers guidance on treatments.
- Looks at evidence.
- Initially claimed to be independent but thought of by some as a government rationing body because NICE evaluates the cost-effectiveness of treatments.
- Has changed advice in response to pressure – flu drugs, hypertension, osteoporosis, dyspepsia.
- Rumours suggest that implementation of NICE guidance will be part of future quality outcomes framework.

CHAPTER 5

CLINICAL GOVERNANCE

The aim of clinical governance is quality assurance, to ensure that medicine is practised to a high and safe standard. A number of concepts, processes and behaviours are required to demonstrate, achieve and maintain a high standard of clinical care. As such, clinical governance issues can arise during the assessment. A good GP should be aware of clinical governance issues and this may be tested during the mock consultations, group discussions and interview.

The following should be implemented:
- Patient and public involvement: what are the public's views and concerns?
- Risk management: includes assessing risk, reporting near misses and significant events, evaluating complaints.
- Clinical audit: evaluating your own practice.
- Clinical effectiveness: including practising evidence-based medicine.
- Staffing and staff management.
- Education and training: continued professional development for doctors, appraisals, courses.

INFORMATION ACCESS AND SHARING

Respect data protection and confidentiality. Caldicott set out a series of principles to guide health-care workers, which are based on the Data Protection Act:

- Justify the purpose for using patient information.
- Do not use personally identifiable information unless absolutely necessary.
- Aim to use the minimum personal identifiable information possible, eg use an identifier number rather than a name.
- Access to patient information should be on a strict need-to-know basis.
- All staff should be aware of their responsibilities to respect patient confidentiality.
- Understand and comply with the law. The most relevant legislation is the Data Protection Act 1998, the Police and Criminal Evidence Act 1984 and the Human Rights Act 1998.

CHAPTER 5

MENTAL CAPACITY ACT 2005

The Mental Capacity Act may be particularly relevant to the mock consultation:

- Came into effect in 2007.
- People can plan their future for a time when they may not have capacity.
- Capacity is decision specific, ie a person cannot be deemed to have a general lack of capacity but capacity will have to be tested against each given situation.
- Decisions should be made in the best interests of the patient. Carers and families should be consulted.
- Restraint may be used if in the person's best interests.
- Lasting Power of Attorney can make health and welfare decisions on behalf of the individual.
- Independent mental capacity advocate (IMCA): someone who is appointed to make representations about the person's wishes, feelings, beliefs and values on behalf of someone who lacks capacity but has no-one to speak on his or her behalf.
- Advance decisions can be made to refuse treatment even if it shortens life. Has to be written, witnessed and signed.
- Ill treatment or neglect of a person who lacks capacity is a criminal offence.
- Research may be carried out involving people who lack capacity if minimal risk and approved by research ethics committee.

CHAPTER 5

Chapter 6
Further Practice
Scenarios

CHAPTER 6

FURTHER PRACTICE SCENARIOS

A good doctor continues to develop, learn and practise his or her technique. The GP VTS assessment is no different. This chapter offers more practice scenarios. Try to go through each question under 'assessment conditions', with a colleague critiquing your performance. Some short notes accompany each scenario; these notes are by no means complete but offer hints for further discussion.

QUESTION 1: A PATIENT WITH DEMENTIA

A 79-year-old man with dementia, attends the surgery with his daughter. She says that he left the gas on last night. What are the issues?

QUESTION 2: A POSSIBLE DIAGNOSIS OF CANCER

A 66-year-old patient comes to the surgery to get her X-ray results, performed for a chronic cough. She stopped smoking 3 years ago. A suspicious looking shadow has been found. How do you manage the consultation?

QUESTION 3: ALTERNATIVE MEDICINE FOR MYELOMA

A patient attends with thoracic back pain, a greatly raised erythrocyte sedimentation rate (ESR) and hypercalcaemia. Protein electrophoresis demonstrates a monoclonal band. Bence Jones proteins have been found in the urine. The patient would like to try yoga rather than conventional medicine as a treatment modality. What do you do?

QUESTION 4: DOCTOR–PATIENT BOUNDARIES

A patient remarks that she would like to have a drink with you. What do you do?

QUESTION 5: BREAKING BAD NEWS (1)

A 32-year-old woman comes to the neurology clinic, anxious to get her results. You have to explain that she has a diagnosis of multiple sclerosis (MS).

QUESTION 6: DEALING WITH OBESITY

A 52-year-old woman presents to the clinic to get her
blood test results. Her thyroid results are normal; you have
to explain that her obesity is caused by a lack of exercise
and poor dietary habits.

QUESTION 7: BREAKING BAD NEWS (2)

A 27-year-old woman has come to the gynaecology clinic. You are to inform her that she is infertile. Previous chlamydia infections, before meeting her current partner, have damaged her fallopian tubes. Swab results are clear of infection.

QUESTION 8: A COLLEAGUE'S MISTAKE

A 70-year-old man comes to your surgery for a well man check. You notice that his prostate-specific antigen or PSA, taken 6 months ago, was raised. A colleague failed to action the result. How do you manage the consultation?

QUESTION 9: DEALING WITH PATIENT DEMANDS

A patient presents with a newspaper cutting of a new drug for obesity. You have never heard of it. The drug costs in excess of £100/month. The patient has not made any effort to lose any weight, but demands that you prescribe the medication. How do you manage the situation?

QUESTION 10: AN INAPPROPRIATE MEMBER OF STAFF

Your practice manager makes inappropriate sexual remarks to you. You hold a meeting with three of your GP colleagues to discuss it. What are the issues? How do you manage the situation?

QUESTION 11: A PATIENT COMPLAINT

A patient attends your clinic claiming that your senior colleague suggested that she should have an internal examination for urinary symptoms. You hold a meeting to discuss this. Your colleague is present, with the nurse manager and the practice manager. What are the issues and how do you manage the situation?

QUESTION 12: A COLLEAGUE'S PERFORMANCE

Your colleague has been treating a patient with thoracic back pain with painkillers and physiotherapy. The patient then sees you in emergency clinic with haemoptysis. You organise a chest X-ray, which shows a suspicious mass and you are concerned that the thoracic pain is secondary to metastases. You refer the patient urgently for investigation. A diagnosis of malignancy is confirmed. This is not the first time that you have been worried about your colleague's performance. What are the issues and how do you manage the situation?

QUESTION 13: PATIENT REGISTRATION

A member of staff asks if her husband can register as a patient. What are the issues?

QUESTION 14: TELEPHONE CONSULTATIONS

The practice manager feels that your practice can be more efficient if doctors and nurses offer a telephone consultation system. You hold a meeting to discuss it. What are the issues?

QUESTION 15: A POORLY PERFORMING NURSE

Your practice nurse is found to have been treating patients with hypertension without involving a GP. She is not a nurse prescriber and has no specialist training in hypertension. What are the issues? How do you manage the situation?

QUESTION 16: PRESSURE FROM THE PCT

The primary care trust (PCT) wants the practice to switch all your patients taking an expensive blood pressure drug to a cheaper generic drug. What are the issues?

QUESTION 17: PRESCRIPTION FRAUD

You caught a patient amending prescriptions to get diazepam. How do you manage the situation?

QUESTION 18: DUTY DOCTOR – GP (1)

You are the on-call doctor at your practice and have just finished morning surgery. There are five duty jobs to do. Put the following in the order that you would deal with them and justify your reasoning:

A   Mr Sanders, COPD, breathless, home visit.

B   Jason Finch, needs another sick note, please call.

C   Sally Williams, needs repeat prescription.

D   Elizabeth Bailey, tearful, please call, stressed.

E   Mark Tucker, has gout again, needs advice.

QUESTION 19: DUTY DOCTOR – GP (2)

You are the on-call doctor at your practice and have just finished morning surgery. There are five duty jobs to do. Put the following in the order that you would deal with them; justify your reasoning:

A   Harry Beale, 87, chest pain.

B   Laurence Booth, 54, chest pain.

C   Joanne Dean, 15, needs morning-after pill a.s.a.p.

D   Anita Winters, 29, severe abdominal pain.

E   Oliver Swain, 5, asthma, wheezing all night.

QUESTION 20: DUTY DOCTOR – GP (3)

You are the on-call doctor at your practice and in the middle of your evening emergency clinic. There are three more patients in the waiting room to see: one with an earache, another with a sore throat and the third with a cough. The receptionist then calls you. A patient has arrived at the practice demanding to see a doctor immediately; he wants his repeat prescription for his blood pressure medication before his holiday tomorrow; he only has 2 days of tablets left and is currently late for a dinner appointment. There is also a phone call to make: 'child with a rash'. In what order do you manage the situation and why?

QUESTION 21: GP – MIDDLE OF THE DAY

You have finished a longer than usual morning surgery. There is a lot of admin work to be done and fortunately there are no jobs on the duty doctor screen. What do you do first and why?

A   Review the day's blood test results.

B   Sign repeat prescriptions.

C   Eat lunch.

D   Read through the day's medical post from the hospital.

E   Dictate referral letters from morning's clinic.

NOTES

QUESTION 1: A PATIENT WITH DEMENTIA

- What other dangerous behaviour has he displayed?
- Is the behaviour new, could there be a reversible cause, such as a urinary tract infection (UTI)?
- Does he live on his own?
- How is his daughter coping?
- Does he have capacity?
- If he doesn't have capacity, consider involving family to do what's in the patient's best interest.

QUESTION 2: A POSSIBLE DIAGNOSIS OF CANCER

- What is the patient concerned about? She may be concerned about cancer, in which case you can say that that might be a possibility. Otherwise, perhaps express your concerns that there is a shadow and ask whether the patient knows what a shadow may be. What are her fears?
- Express that the shadow ought to be checked out. Is it ok for a referral to be made? Does she know what to expect? Does she have any questions?
- Would she like to come back, perhaps with a relative, once she has had a chance to think about what's happened?

QUESTION 3: ALTERNATIVE MEDICINE FOR MYELOMA

- Does the patient understand that she has a diagnosis of multiple myeloma?
- Does she realise that it is a malignant disease?
- Does she understand the consequences of not having treatment?

QUESTION 4: DOCTOR–PATIENT BOUNDARIES

- The General Medical Council (GMC) has clear guidance on this. Simply, the answer is no.
- What is the effect on the doctor–patient relationship?
- Remember to ask for a chaperone for your own protection if an intimate clinical examination is required.
- How will you manage future consultations?

QUESTION 5: BREAKING BAD NEWS (1)

- Does she know what the tests were for?
- Does she want to bring any family members in with her?
- Break bad news with empathy.
- What does she know about MS?
- What are her fears?
- Does she have questions: about treatment, outlook for the future, what next, will it affect fertility?

QUESTION 6: DEALING WITH OBESITY

- Explain that the thyroid results are normal.
- Does she have any idea as to why she is overweight?
- Ask her about lifestyle habits: what does she think about her lifestyle? Are there any aspects of her lifestyle that she could change?
- Does she think that her lifestyle has caused her to put on weight?
- Health promotion: does she smoke? What are her cardiac risk factors? Should her cholesterol and glucose be checked?

CONSULTATION NOTES

QUESTION 7: BREAKING BAD NEWS (2)

- Confirm patient identity.
- If with her partner, explain that you would like to see her alone for a moment. Establish whether her partner knows about the history of chlamydia infection.
- Ask that patient what she knows so far and what her concerns are. You may just need to confirm her fears.
- Break the bad news; explain that infection can damage the tubes.
- What are her views?
- Explain that she does not have the infection any more.
- Give hope: options for fertility treatment need to be discussed.

QUESTION 8: A COLLEAGUE'S MISTAKE

- Check if the patient was referred to the hospital recently; it may be the referral was not entered into the patient's records.
- Is the patient aware that a PSA test was done 6 months ago?
- Apologise for any oversight.
- Explain that an urgent referral will be made.
- Understand the patient's anger.
- Explain that you will investigate what happened, eg discuss with the doctor concerned.

QUESTION 9: DEALING WITH PATIENT DEMANDS

- Is the drug safe? What are the guidelines surrounding its use?
- Why has the patient not made an effort to lose weight? Is the patient depressed?
- Can you justify spending that money on a patient who is not helping herself?
- Will the patient see prescribing the drug a mandate to continue an unhealthy lifestyle?
- Are there other ways you can help the patient lose weight?
- You are not obliged to prescribe the drug.

QUESTION 10: AN INAPPROPRIATE MEMBER OF STAFF

- Has she done this before?
- How did it make you feel?
- Explain to her that you felt that her behaviour was inappropriate and you would like it to stop.
- If further episodes occur, consider disciplinary action. Discuss with employment law advisers, local medical committee (LMC) or the British Medical Association (BMA).

GROUP NOTES

QUESTION 11: A PATIENT COMPLAINT

- This is a potentially serious situation.
- Explain to your senior colleague what has happened and that a meeting needs to be held. Do not be judgemental.
- Review the patient's record: what were the patient's symptoms? Did they warrant an intimate exam? Did your colleague offer a chaperone?
- Was there a misunderstanding and lack of communication? Was the doctor concerned about a sexually transmitted infection or STI and did he feel that vaginal swabs should be taken?
- Should your colleague be offered time off pending an investigation?
- What could be done to avoid the same situation happening again?

QUESTION 12: A COLLEAGUE'S PERFORMANCE

- Explain to your colleague what has happened and what other concerns you have.
- Review the notes of the patient in question. Has the patient's health suffered as a consequence of your colleague's management?
- Do all of the doctor's patient's records need to be reviewed?
- Consider performance managing the doctor.
- Does the doctor have problems: depression, drugs or alcohol? Can you help with these?
- What advice does your medical defence union or the GMC offer?

QUESTION 13: PATIENT REGISTRATION

- Will the husband expect preferential treatment?
- Can the practice offer impartial care?
- The member of staff may need to handle her husband's medical records. Confidentiality may be compromised.
- Will other staff members expect their families to be allowed registration with the practice?

QUESTION 14: TELEPHONE CONSULTATIONS

- Why do they think that a telephone system is required?
- How can the practitioner confirm the identity of the caller?
- Is training required in telephone consulting?
- It is hard to assess patients over the phone. What failsafe systems will be put in place to ensure against clinical mishaps?
- Is it more efficient than face-to face consulting?
- Will you need to increase you medical indemnity insurance cover?

GROUP NOTES

QUESTION 15: A POORLY PERFORMING NURSE

- All her patients need to be reviewed.
- Have there been any other clinical concerns?
- Have there been adverse events as a result of her management? Affected patients may need to be recalled.
- Has she been signing prescriptions? This is unlawful given that she is not a nurse prescriber.
- Make the nurse aware of your concern as soon as possible.
- What are her views?
- Seek advice from the BMA/LMC/Nursing and Midwifery Council (NMC).
- Disciplinary action/dismissible offence?

QUESTION 16: PRESSURE FROM THE PCT

- Is there evidence that the drug is as effective as the more expensive one, with no more side effects or interactions?
- Is the drug in the same class as the more expensive one?
- Is it reasonable, given the current NHS crisis?
- How will you inform patients of the change?
- Is it safe to change all drugs in a batch or will each case need to be reviewed?
- Who will change the drugs? Will the PCT pay the practice money for the hours of work required?

GROUP NOTES

QUESTION 17: PRESCRIPTION FRAUD

- This is a criminal offence and the police should be involved.
- All doctors in the practice, local practices and pharmacies, and the PCT should be informed.
- Does the patient have an illness that requires medical help, eg anxiety?

QUESTION 18: DUTY DOCTOR – GP (1)

Suggested answer: A C D E B

Mr Sanders ought to be called first to ensure that his situation is not serious. If it is, a home visit or emergency ambulance may need to be arranged. A repeat prescription may be for something simple like the contraceptive pill, or Sally Williams may be calling for more inhalers because her asthma has deteriorated and she is very breathless. Elizabeth Bailey may be stressed and could be at risk of self-harm. Gout and another sick certificate are not life threatening.

QUESTION 19: DUTY DOCTOR – GP (2)

Suggested answer: E B D A C

As long as your answers are justified with good reasoning, they are acceptable. Asthma has a significant mortality. The child has been wheezing all night and could be tired and at risk of respiratory arrest. Mr Booth and Mr Beale may be having cardiac events. Mr Booth is young and ought to be called next. If his features are of concern, you may elect to arrange an emergency ambulance. Mr Beale is 87; he again may be having a cardiac event but Anita Winters is young and may have an ectopic pregnancy. Both warrant urgent reviews. Can you ask for help and delegate some tasks to your colleagues? If not, Anita should be called followed by Mr Beale. Although Joanne Dean may or may not be at the end of the 72-hour window for the morning-after pill, her condition is life changing but not life threatening.

QUESTION 20: DUTY DOCTOR – GP (3)

This is a difficult situation because you may not know exactly how unwell the patients in the waiting room are. Is it possible to ask a colleague to deal with the phone call? If not, perhaps eyeball the patients in the waiting room to check if they look sick or well. The patient with the earache may be febrile and vomiting. The patient with the sore throat may be septic and drooling with a peritonsillar abscess and the patient with the cough could be in respiratory distress. Take a moment to announce that you have an urgent phone call to make. You may ask the parents to bring the child with the rash to the clinic straight away or indeed to call an ambulance. The patients in the waiting room are there for medical reasons and should be managed first. Only then should the man demanding the prescription be dealt with.

QUESTION 21: GP – MIDDLE OF THE DAY

Suggested answer: C E A B D

It is important to look after your own health, to wind down and recharge with lunch. Dictating the referral letters with the patients fresh in your mind will make life easier and also help the secretary keep on top of her work, rather than getting a dictation tape late in the day. Although most hospital laboratories ring GP practices with any results of concern, it is best to go through them to ensure that no urgent action is required. Signing the prescriptions next means that the patients can get their drugs on time. Hospital letters tend to arrive a few weeks after patients have been seen in clinic. They may require actions and should be read regularly.

PRIORITISATION NOTES

Appendices

APPENDIX A
COMMONLY USED TERMS

A&E	accident and emergency
ABPM	ambulatory blood pressure monitor
ADHD	attention deficit hyperactivity disorder
AF	atrial fibrillation
AS	aortic stenosis
ASs	additional services: services such as child health surveillance, contraception and cervical screening, ie services that GPs routinely provide at present
AV	atrioventricular
BMI	body mass index
BP	blood pressure
CF	cystic fibrosis
CHAI	Commission for Health Audit and Inspection
CHI	Commission for Health Improvement: has responsibility for ensuring that government set health policies and National Service Frameworks (NSFs), along with clinical guidance issued by NICE, are met. Reviews are carried out every 3–4 years as standard. CHI is also involved in the investigation and enquiries of serious service failures. Website: www.chi.nhs.uk
CNS	central nervous system
COC	combined oral contraceptive
COPD	chronic obstructive pulmonary disease
DENs	doctor's educational needs

DESs	directed enhanced services: special services provided locally by GPs that have been negotiated nationally. All practices can choose whether to provide these services. New DESs were introduced in 2006–07 and were carried over to 2007–08. These services are more specialised and, although the PCO is expected to ensure provision of these services, not all practices will offer everything
DKA	diabetic ketoacidosis
DVT	deep vein thrombosis
ECG	electrocardiogram
ENT	ear, nose and throat
FBC	full blood count
FRC	functional residual capacity
GI	gastrointestinal
GMC	General Medical Council: the GMC registers all doctors practising in the UK and regulates and promotes good medical practice and behaviour. Website: www.gmc-uk.org
GMS contract	General Medical Services contract: national contract between GP practices and PCOs to provide primary care services to their local communities. May also be referred to as new GMS
GP ST	General Practice Speciality Training
GP VTS	General Practice Vocational Training Scheme; alternative name for GP Speciality Training
GPwSI	general practitioner with a special interest
GTN	glyceryl trinitrate
GUM	genitourinary medicine
HbA1c	glycated haemoglobin
HCA	health-care assistant
HCHS	hospital and community health services: the main elements of these are the provision of hospital services and certain community health services, such as district nursing. These services are provided in the main by NHS trusts

HIV	human immunodeficiency virus
HRT	hormone replacement therapy
ICU	intensive care unit
IMCA	independent mental capacity advocate
JCPTGP	Joint Committee on Postgraduate Training for General Practice: since 2005 responsibility has passed to PMETB
LES	local enhanced service: tailored to local needs
LFTs	liver function tests
LMC	local medical committee
MI	myocardial infarction
MMR	measles, mumps and rubella
MRCGP	membership of the Royal College of General Practitioners
MRI	magnetic resonance imaging
NatPaCT	National Primary and Care Trust: although the NatPaCT development programme is no longer running. The website is a good source of information on GPwSi, clinical audit and LES. Website: www.natpact.nhs.uk
NCAS	National Clinical Assessment Service: part of the NPSA (see below), it provides confidential advice and support to the NHS when the performance of a doctor gives cause for concern. Website: www.ncaa.nhs.uk
NES	national enhanced services: the PCO will decide whether to provide these services.
nGMS contract	new General Medical Services contract
NICE	National Institute for Health and Clinical Excellence: a national, independent organisation that provides guidance on ill health and associated treatments and promoting good health. Website: www.nice.org.uk
NNH	number needed to harm

NNT	number needed to treat
NPS	national person specification: a list of competencies used to assess suitability for a career in general practice. Website: www.gprecruitment.org.uk
NPSA	National Patient Safety Agency: the NPSA is a special health authority created in July 2001 to coordinate the efforts of the entire country to report, and more importantly to learn from, adverse events occurring in the NHS
OCD	obsessive–compulsive disorder
OOHs	out-of-hours services: 18:30–8:00 on weekdays and all weekends and bank holidays, when care can be provided by doctors from a number of different surgeries, or by private companies
PBC	practice-based commissioning
PCC	primary care contracting: provides support for commissioners. Information on quality outcomes framework and primary care service frameworks. Website: www.primarycarecontracting.nhs.uk
PCO	primary care organisation: responsible for the management of independent primary care contractors, eg PCTs
PCT	primary care trust: responsible for the planning and securing of health services, and for improving the health of the local population. Since April 2002, 303 PCTs took over the responsibility (from health authorities) for planning and commissioning local health services. Over time PCTs will become responsible for the control of 75% of the NHS budget
PEC	professional executive committee: leads and guides the PCT
PEFR	peak expiratory flow rate
PMETB	postgraduate medical education and training board: independent body responsible for GP training in the UK. Website: www.pmetb.org.uk

PMS	personal medical service; a PMS contract is an alternative to the GMS contract, and very specific to the local community
POP	progestogen-only pill
PUNs	patient's unmet needs
QALY	quality-adjusted life-year
QOF	quality and outcomes framework: additional funding stream for the practice generated via attainment of points through clinical and non-clinical domains
RA	rheumatoid arthritis
RCGP	Royal College of General Practitioners. Website: www.rcgp.org.uk
RCT	randomised controlled trial
RICE	rest, ice, compression and elevation
SHAs	strategic health authorities: an April 2002 28 SHAs took over from the pre-existing 95 English health authorities. They are responsible for developing strategies for local health services and ensuring high-quality performance.
SIFT	service increment for teaching: medical student support, formerly service increment for teaching (SIFT), is a special NHS levy that is given out as extra funds to NHS institutions participating in training undergraduate students. It covers the costs to the NHS of supporting the teaching of medical undergraduates. It is not a payment for teaching as such, eg consultants in an outpatient clinic or a GP in a surgery generally see fewer patients if students are present. SIFT is intended to meet this sort of excess cost, rather than pass it on to health-care purchasers
SSRI	selective serotonin release inhibitor
STI	sexually transmitted infection
T_4	thyroxine
TB	tuberculosis
TED	thromboembolic deterrent

TFT	thyroid function test
TIA	transient ischaemic attack
TSH	thyroid-stimulating hormone
UTI	urinary tract infection
URTI	upper respiratory tract infection
WCC	white cell count

APPENDIX B
REFERENCES

Eve R (2003). *PUNs and DENs: Discovering Learning Needs in General Practice*. Oxford: Radcliffe Publishing Ltd.

Luft J (1961). The Johari window. *Human Relations Training News* 5.1: 6–7.

Luft J (1969). *Of Human Interaction*. Palo Alto, CA: National Press.

Luft J, Ingham H (1955). *The Johari Window: A graphic model for interpersonal relations*. University Of California Western Training Lab.

Neighbour R (2004). *The Inner Consultation*, 2nd edn. Oxford: Radcliffe Publishing Ltd.

Pendleton D, Schofield T, Tate P and Havelock P (2003). *The New Consultation*, 2nd edn. Oxford: Oxford University Press.

Prochaska J, DiClemente C (1983). Stages and processes of self-change of smoking: towards an integrated model of change. *J Consulting Clin Psychol* 51: 390–5.

INDEX